Building Health Promotion Capacity

*Scott McLean, Joan Feather,
and David Butler-Jones*

Building Health Promotion Capacity: Action for Learning, Learning from Action

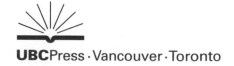

UBCPress · Vancouver · Toronto

15 14 13 12 11 10 09 08 07 06 05   5 4 3 2 1

Printed in Canada on acid-free paper

Library and Archives Canada Cataloguing in Publication

McLean, Scott, 1965-
   Building health promotion capacity : action for learning, learning from action /
Scott McLean, Joan Feather, and David Butler-Jones.

Includes bibliographical references and index.
ISBN 0-7748-1150-1

   1. Health promotion. 2. Public health. 3. Health promotion – Saskatchewan.
4. Health education – Saskatchewan. I. Feather, Joan, 1944- II. Butler-Jones, David.
III. Title.

RA427.8.M395 2005   613   C2004-906769-9

Canadä

UBC Press gratefully acknowledges the financial support for our publishing program of the Government of Canada through the Book Publishing Industry Development Program (BPIDP), and of the Canada Council for the Arts, and the British Columbia Arts Council.

This book has been published with the help of a grant from the Saskatchewan Heart Health Program.

Printed and bound in Canada by Friesens
Set in Stone by Artegraphica Design Co. Ltd.
Copy editor: Francis Chow
Proofreader: Kate Spezowka
Indexer: Patricia Buchanan

UBC Press
The University of British Columbia
2029 West Mall
Vancouver, BC V6T 1Z2
604-822-5959 / Fax: 604-822-6083
www.ubcpress.ca

Contents

Tables and Figures

Acknowledgments

This book is the result of substantial work on the part of many people beyond its three co-authors. We would like to thank the staff members who served the Building Health Promotion Capacity (BHPC) project over its five years of operation (1998-2003): Georgia Bell-Woodard (September 1999 through 2003), Lori Ebbesen, Lorraine Khatchatourians (December 1998 through 2003), Meredith Moore, Karen Schmidt, Bonnie Sproat (to December 1998), and Sheilagh Steer (to June 1999).

These individuals made many contributions to this book. They developed, delivered, and evaluated the capacity-building interventions described in Chapter 4. They gathered and analyzed much of the data whose synthesis is presented in Chapters 5 through 7. They, along with our co-investigators Kathryn Green, Bruce Reeder, and Sheilagh Steer, provided feedback on numerous drafts of this book.

Lori Ebbesen had a distinctive role in the development of research instruments and processes, in the collection of data, and in the initial interpretation of such data. Meredith Moore and Georgia Bell-Woodard had distinctive roles in the organization of capacity-building interventions and in the interpretation of what was learned from such interventions. Karen Schmidt provided excellent administrative support to the BHPC program, while Lorraine Khatchatourians and Bonnie Sproat developed and facilitated the HPLINK listserv.

We gratefully acknowledge the funding provided by the National Health Research and Development Program, the Canadian Institutes of Health Research, Saskatchewan Health, and the Heart and Stroke Foundation of Saskatchewan. In addition to financial support, Saskatchewan Health and the Heart and Stroke Foundation of Saskatchewan were key partners in our program of intervention and research, providing important advice and human resources for our work.

This book is based on extensive involvement with many willing and dedicated health and human service workers in the province of Saskatchewan, to whom we owe our thanks. Such people served our project in many roles: as participants, educators, and facilitators in our interventions; as respondents and participants in our research processes; and as readers and commentators on our evolving ideas about health promotion capacity and its development. We extend our appreciation to all those who took part in our capacity-building and research practices.

Abbreviations

BHPC   Building Health Promotion Capacity
CHHI   Canadian Heart Health Initiative
HPC   Health Promotion Contact
NHRDP   National Health Research and Development Program
PRHPRC   Prairie Region Health Promotion Research Centre
SAHO   Saskatchewan Association of Health Organizations
SHHP   Saskatchewan Heart Health Program
SPHPP   Saskatchewan Population Health Promotion Partnership

Part 1
Setting the Stage

1

Introduction: Action, Learning, and Capacity Building

In this book, we explore how individuals become more effective in health promotion work, and how organizations become more effective in supporting such work. The first stage of this exploration is about "action for learning." To take action for learning is to do something to influence the knowledge, skills, or dispositions of oneself or others. In this book, we narrate how we took action to facilitate the learning of practitioners and leaders in the field of health promotion. To take action for learning is to hope that "learning from action" will occur. To learn from action is to change oneself as a result of experience and subsequent reflection on that experience. Here we narrate what we learned about health promotion capacity and its development by taking action to facilitate the learning of practitioners and leaders in that field.

The concept of "capacity" structures our exploration of action and learning. In simple terms, capacity refers to those qualities or characteristics that enable people to do something. Given the social nature of human life, the capacity to act is not determined solely by the qualities and characteristics of the individual person. Rather, the individual's capacity to act is mediated by the environment in which he or she acts. When looking at capacity for complex professional practices such as those related to health promotion, we see that the environment typically entails both an immediate organizational setting within which individuals work and a broader social context within which both the individual and his or her organization exist. Building capacity means developing the qualities and characteristics of the individual, and shaping the organizational and social environment within which that individual will act.

This book is based on the experiences of the Building Health Promotion Capacity (BHPC) project from 1998 to 2003. BHPC was also known as the dissemination research phase of the Saskatchewan Heart Health

Program. BHPC was an applied research project designed to enhance the capacity of practitioners and regional health districts in Saskatchewan to undertake effective health promotion activities, and to develop an understanding of capacity and capacity building. Taking action for learning and learning from action represent our fundamental approach to building health promotion capacity.

Outline

We explore action, learning, and capacity building through seven chapters. Chapter 2 provides contextual and conceptual background to the action and learning described in subsequent chapters. Chapter 2 locates our work in a historical and theoretical context, and describes how we organized ourselves to undertake this work. We describe the evolution of public policies and health reforms in Saskatchewan during the late 1900s. We then describe the origins of the BHPC project, through a description of the Saskatchewan Heart Health Program and related efforts to support and enhance the population health promotion work of regional health districts across the province. We then locate our work within existing models of health promotion and the dissemination of capacity.

Chapters 3 and 4 examine the ways in which we took action for learning. We acted in order to build our understanding of the processes through which capacity can be built among individuals and organizations involved in health promotion work. We designed a series of research activities to gain a better understanding of the evolution of capacity for health promotion in Saskatchewan. In Chapter 3, we describe our six research methods: (1) surveys and interviews with practitioners and health district leaders, (2) key informant interviews, (3) case studies, (4) think tanks, (5) evaluation research, and (6) participant observation. These research methods were designed to help us learn about health promotion capacity and its development.

We also acted in order to facilitate the learning of others. We designed a series of interventions to enhance the knowledge, skills, and commitment of key health promotion actors across Saskatchewan. In Chapter 4, we describe our six forms of intervention: (1) delivering an annual health promotion summer school, (2) organizing regional and provincial continuing education events, (3) facilitating an Internet-based listserv, (4) nurturing relationships with health promotion practitioners, (5) advocating for population health promotion among health district leaders, and (6) providing consulting services and support to existing networks. These interventions were designed to help health promotion practitioners and health district leaders better understand, embrace, and implement population health promotion activities. Although separated into different chapters, our two modes of taking action for learning were integrated both conceptually and in practice. Doing research was in part a capacity-building intervention, and doing capacity building was in part a means to learn about capacity and its development.

Chapters 5 through 7 examine the learning we accomplished through our continuing education and research activities. Chapter 5 explores what we learned about health promotion capacity among individual practitioners. We assert that individuals' health promotion capacity consists of four elements: knowledge, skills, commitment, and resources. We argue that practitioners' health promotion capacity is enhanced through four key catalysts: (1) support from managers and colleagues, (2) new roles and responsibilities, (3) opportunities to encounter new ideas and practices, and (4) opportunities to apply new knowledge and skills. The catalysts to greater individual health promotion capacity are rooted in the organizational and environmental context within which individuals work.

Chapter 6 explores what we learned about health promotion capacity among organizations. We assert that organizations' health promotion capacity consists of four elements: commitment, culture, structures, and resources. We argue that organizations' health promotion capacity is enhanced through seven key catalysts: (1) opportunities to work on meaningful projects and partnerships, (2) access to health promotion resources, (3) systematic planning and evaluation exercises, (4) individual capacity building, (5) changes to key personnel, (6) organizational restructuring, and (7) the strategic actions of change agents. The catalysts to greater organizational capacity to support health promotion work are rooted in part in the activities of individuals who contribute to organizations, and in part in the environment in which such organizations exist.

Chapter 7 explores what we learned about the influence of the environment on the health promotion capacity of individual practitioners and regional health districts. We argue that four environmental factors are particularly influential in supporting or hindering the capacity of individuals and organizations to engage in health promotion work: political will, public opinion, supportive organizations, and ideas and other resources. The relationship between these factors and health promotion capacity is not unidirectional. Through activities such as advocacy, political action, and research, individuals and organizations may influence the nature of the environment within which they engage in health promotion work.

Chapter 8 synthesizes the major insights of our work and proposes a number of conclusions. We summarize the nature of health promotion capacity by presenting checklists that identify the elements of individual and organizational capacity and the characteristics of environments supportive of such capacity. We summarize the nature of capacity development by reviewing the key catalysts of capacity for individuals and organizations. We conclude by outlining the key implications of our findings for practitioners, leaders, policy makers, and scholars, both within health promotion and in other fields.

Conclusion

While this book is grounded in the practice of health promotion in Saskatchewan, its insights are transferable to many other places and domains of professional practice. The nature and development of health promotion capacity in Saskatchewan contains lessons of use to those interested in health promotion capacity across Canada and beyond. While the geographic scope of our research was limited to one Canadian province, the implications of our findings are important to many other places.

Our book resonates with fields of professional practice outside the realm of health promotion. The nature of capacity among individuals and organizations engaged in health promotion work is not radically different from that among individuals and organizations engaged in substantive fields such as social work, adult education, community development, and regional or urban planning. While readers interested in these and other fields may define the elements of capacity somewhat differently, they will recognize obvious parallels in terms of what constitutes capacity and how capacity is developed.

Our book also has insights of value to scholars and practitioners in continuing professional education, human resource development, and organizational development. Even in fields where the content of capacity for good professional practice may be dramatically different from that of health promotion, the process of capacity development is roughly parallel. The methods through which we have defined capacity and identified the key catalysts to the development of capacity are applicable to continuing professional educators and organizational developers in many fields.

The application of our concepts and methods to other places and domains of professional practice should be fruitful for many readers.

We have therefore written this book to be accessible not only to readers interested in health promotion but also to those in related fields. We have endeavoured to balance the interests of practitioners, leaders, policy makers, and scholars. In practical terms, this means that we have used accessible language, incorporated only a modest amount of empirical data, and consolidated references to scholarly literature in Chapter 2.

2

Making the Building Health Promotion Capacity Project Happen

This chapter provides the context of the Building Health Promotion Capacity (BHPC) project. We describe the social and public policy context for health promotion in Saskatchewan in the late twentieth century. We then describe how we came together as a team, how we mobilized the resources required to do our work, and how we structured our efforts to do that work. Finally, we locate our action and learning in evolving discourses on health promotion and capacity building.

A Context for Action (I):
Saskatchewan in the Late Twentieth Century

While popular images and many public institutions in Saskatchewan are still oriented toward a rural way of life, the province is no longer an agrarian society. Changes in demographic, economic, and community structures have all been important in recent decades. Demographically, Saskatchewan has experienced significant net out-migration, movement from farms to cities, an aging of the population, and strong growth in the Aboriginal population (Saskatchewan Bureau of Statistics 1995). Economic production and employment have shifted away from agriculture and toward the service sector. In terms of community structure, there has been substantial urbanization, with people, businesses, employers, and services becoming increasingly concentrated in a relatively small number of urban centres (Stabler, Olfert, and Fulton 1992).

On the one hand, it is possible to paint a rather negative picture of Saskatchewan in the late twentieth century. External factors seemed to be at the root of hard times: technological change and declining terms of trade for agricultural commodities made it impossible to sustain the demographic, economic, and community structures of Saskatchewan's agrarian past. On the other hand, people in Saskatchewan enjoyed a very high quality of life. Using the United Nations' human development indicators (average levels of education, life expectancy, and income), Saskatchewan consistently came out near the top in comparisons with other Canadian provinces. Saskatchewan enjoyed high levels of volunteerism and collective action. The province had a remarkable density of cooperatives, local governments, mutual support groups, and other community-based organizations (Simbandumwe, Fulton, and Hammond Ketilson 1991; Miller, Miller, and McLean 1996). Through thousands of such organizations, Saskatchewan had a tremendous human resource of people experienced in voluntary and collective action, and committed to building healthy and sustainable communities.

Public Policy and Health Reform

A community-based approach to social change was a hallmark of public policy in Saskatchewan during the 1990s. The centrality of community-based approaches to public sector challenges can be perceived in titles of public policy statements issued by a range of provincial departments:

- *Working Together Toward Wellness: A Saskatchewan Vision for Health* (Saskatchewan Health 1992)
- *Report of the Minister's Advisory Committee on Inter-Community Co-operation and Community Quality of Life* (Saskatchewan Municipal Government 1993)
- *Responding to the Community: Proposals for Cultural Development* (Saskatchewan Municipal Government 1995)
- *Regional Economic Development Authorities: Building Capacity and Sharing Responsibility in Community-Based Economic Development* (Saskatchewan Economic Development 1995)
- *Saskatchewan Human Services: Working with Communities* (Saskatchewan Human Services Integration Forum 2000)
- *School Plus. A Vision for Children and Youth: The Final Report of the Task Force and Public Dialogue on the Role of the School: Toward a New School, Community and Human Service Partnership in Saskatchewan* (Saskatchewan Education 2001)

The resurgence of community-based approaches to the provision of government services was particularly evident in the field of health. Saskatchewan Health (1992, 11) elaborated four key principles of its "wellness approach" to health care:

- create a health system that is responsive to community needs by placing control and management responsibilities at a local level;
- balance the health system's current focus on treatment by emphasizing disease and accident prevention, consumer information, health education, health promotion and early intervention;
- eliminate inequities in the health system by responding to the needs of women, families, the elderly, persons with low incomes, and others with special health needs; and
- make the health system more effective and efficient by integrating institutional, community-based and preventive programs, and by reducing waste and unnecessary duplication at all levels.

In terms of public policy, the wellness model of the 1990s provided much clearer support for health promotion practices than did public policies in Saskatchewan during the 1980s (Feather 1994a; Saskatchewan Health, Population Health Branch 1999).

Health Districts
During the 1980s, several studies as well as prominent agencies recommended the decentralization and devolution of health care planning and decision making. There were several reasons for this, including: (1) a recognition that the health care system was fragmented and uncoordinated, (2) the need to cut costs, (3) a recognition that health status was not directly related to funding and that there were continued inequities in health status, (4) a greater awareness of the determinants of health, and (5) the desire for greater public involvement. In 1992, health reform resulted in the creation of a health district system. Between 1993 and 2002, thirty-two health districts provided a broad range of health services (generally excluding physician services) across Saskatchewan. Several hundred previously existing hospital, home care, and public health boards were dissolved when they were replaced by the district boards. Governing boards of health districts were made up of appointed and elected members.

Health district boards received the vast majority of their operational funding from the provincial government under policies that initially allowed transfer of funds from the acute care sector to the community sector, but not the reverse. The personnel and financial resources of districts were quite variable and reflected the population level of the district as well as the extent to which acute care services were provided. For example, the Saskatoon and Regina Health Districts, each with populations greater than 200,000, had correspondingly large acute care and community service components, and provided the majority of the province's tertiary care services. At the other end of the spectrum, sixteen of the districts had populations under 20,000.

The wellness approach on which district formation was based had health promotion and disease prevention as key strategies. Health promotion meant not only education but also training, research, and community development, while prevention focused on reducing or eliminating the causes of illness or injury. Public health was integrated into the health districts along with other community health services, including mental health, nutrition, and addiction services. Although these services came into the district system relatively late – several years after the integration of hospitals, long-term care, home care, and emergency services – by 1996 all districts had public health services as an integral part of their service array.

At the same time, the concept of population health promotion was gaining currency. For example, a working group formed to help districts improve community services reported in 1998 on the changing role of public health nurses. It outlined the need to confront challenges involved in shifting public health nursing practice from a focus on health education and clinical services to a broader responsibility for population health promotion using strategies such as community development and advocacy. It recognized that the provincial government and the health districts would have to invest in a professional development strategy to ensure that public health and other staff had the competencies necessary for this expanded role.

By the late 1990s, it was clear that further changes were needed to ensure a sustainable, publicly funded, and publicly administered health system. The report of the Commission on Medicare (2001), headed by Ken Fyke, and a subsequent action plan announced by Saskatchewan Health (2002) proposed consolidation of the thirty-two health districts into twelve regional health authorities, with appointed boards and a greater emphasis on primary health services. Population health promotion would continue to be an important function of the regions, with the province playing a larger role in province-wide initiatives. Reorganization of the districts into regions was completed in late 2002.

A Context for Action (II):
National and Provincial Heart Health Movements
Provincial health reforms provided a fundamental impetus for our work in the BHPC project. The transformation of the provincial health system

toward a regionally devolved wellness model of health care created evident and abundant needs for individual learning and organizational development. Health districts became the key organizations in this emerging system, and so we believed that building the health promotion capacity of health districts would be an effective and sustainable contribution to the health of the people of Saskatchewan.

National resources for making this contribution were obtained through participation in the Canadian Heart Health Initiative (CHHI). CHHI was a unique collaboration between Health Canada, provincial departments of health, and the academic and nonprofit sectors (Health and Welfare Canada 1992a; Stachenko 1996). In most provinces, CHHI evolved through three phases: heart health surveys, community demonstration projects, and dissemination research. In addition to its work across Canada, CHHI was influential in major international cardiovascular disease prevention initiatives, including the organization of heart health conferences in Victoria, Barcelona, Singapore, Osaka, and Milan (Advisory Board 1992, 1995, 1998, 2001, 2004).

The Saskatchewan Heart Health Program (SHHP) evolved in phases comparable to those of the other provinces. In the first phase (1989-90), the Saskatchewan Heart Health Survey provided epidemiological data concerning risk factors for cardiovascular disease (Reeder 1990, 1996; Brunt et al. 1995). In the second phase (1992-96), community demonstration projects were undertaken in Regina and the Coteau Hills region. The community demonstration phase of SHHP was jointly funded by Health Canada, Saskatchewan Health, and the Heart and Stroke Foundation of Saskatchewan, and its headquarters were at the Department of Community Health and Epidemiology at the University of Saskatchewan.

The overall objectives of the SHHP demonstration phase were to: (1) reduce the prevalence of risk factors for cardiovascular and related chronic diseases; (2) promote the reduction of socioeconomic, demographic, geographic, and gender risk factor inequity related to cardiovascular disease; and (3) increase the understanding and use of effective strategies for health promotion and prevention of cardiovascular and related chronic diseases. The demonstration phase generated substantial insight into processes of heart health promotion, including: (1) building provincial and local coalitions, (2) community-based programming and advocacy for risk factor reduction, and (3) encouraging the formation of networks among professionals interested in heart health promotion. More detailed information concerning the objectives, structure, and history of the demonstration phase is available in Ebbesen, Rutherford, and

Reeder 1996; Ebbesen et al. 1996; Saskatchewan Heart Health Coalition 1997; and Saskatchewan Heart Health Program 1998a, 1998b, 1998c, 1998d.

Making Action Possible: Building a Team, a Focus, and a Resource Base
The BHPC project became a reality due to the convergence of the two contextual developments described in this chapter so far. The first was the evolution of provincial policies and administrative structures to address population health promotion in Saskatchewan. The second was the transition of SHHP following the completion of its community demonstration projects. In 1996, the principal investigators of the SHHP demonstration phase (Dr. Bruce Reeder and Dr. David Butler-Jones) convened a series of meetings involving SHHP employees, representatives of the Heart and Stroke Foundation of Saskatchewan (HSFS) and Saskatchewan Health, and University of Saskatchewan faculty members to explore a "dissemination phase" for SHHP.

The focus of the SHHP dissemination research phase (known in this book by the more descriptive and succinct acronym BHPC) was constructed at the intersection of Saskatchewan Health's interest in capacity building for population health promotion and the interest of the heart health movement in learning from such processes of capacity building. The BHPC project moved cardiovascular disease prevention solidly into population health promotion terrain, and examined the role of individual learning and organizational development in the dissemination of capacities that would contribute to a reduction of cardiovascular disease. This convergence of interest was made concrete in our successful funding proposals to three agencies: Saskatchewan Health, the Heart and Stroke Foundation of Saskatchewan, and the National Health Research and Development Program (NHRDP; subsequently part of the Canadian Institutes for Health Research). Each of these agencies contributed stable five-year funding to the BHPC project. The total amount funded was just under $1.3 million, with approximately half from NHRDP, somewhat over one-quarter from Saskatchewan Health, and somewhat less than one-quarter from the Heart and Stroke Foundation of Saskatchewan.

To implement the BHPC project, the principal investigators (Dr. Scott McLean and Dr. David Butler-Jones) contracted the services of the Prairie Region Health Promotion Research Centre (PRHPRC). For several previous years, PRHPRC and Saskatchewan Health's Population Health Branch had collaborated on initiatives to provide health promotion training and resource development for practitioners in public and nongovernmental agencies. The centre had organized continuing education events and published resource material in areas such as integrating community development approaches in needs assessment processes (Feather, McGowan, and Moore 1994), using tools and methods for reflective health promotion practice (Feather and Labonte 1995), and applying key concepts in health promotion practice (Kuyek and Labonte 1995; Feather and Sproat 1996). It had become well known among health promotion practitioners and organizations in Saskatchewan, and was looked to for advice, training, and information.

The BHPC project was managed by PRHPRC, with Joan Feather as project coordinator. She assembled a team consisting of a full-time administrative/clerical assistant, a full-time research officer, two part-time program officers, and a part-time communications assistant. This team held monthly action planning and reflection meetings, and used a flexible system of subteams for specific projects. The team operationalized our mission and objectives. Interaction between investigators and staff continued throughout the program, with regular retreats and open communication.

Situating Action in Discourse: Conceptual Foundations of BHPC
BHPC was characterized by two fundamental assumptions that distinguished our efforts from many previous "heart health" projects. First, we believed that a disease-specific approach to health promotion would be less effective than a population-based approach. It is for this reason that our work virtually never mentioned cardiovascular disease, but rather focused attention on addressing the "upstream" determinants of health that predispose people to suffering from heart disease and stroke, among a range of other health problems. It is also for this reason that we regarded the skills and knowledge required for heart health promotion as generic capacities that, if fully developed, would enable organizations, practitioners, and communities to address any of the conditions affecting health, according to local priorities.

Second, we believed that making changes to the determinants of the health of populations requires sustained and strategic action by individuals and organizations having significant capacity to work with communities. For this reason, our work did not attempt to either transfer programmatic initiatives or resources to practitioners or directly reach those who were suffering from or who were at risk of cardiovascular disease. Rather, we strategically invested the resources at our disposal to nurture a learning community among health promotion practitioners and leaders, with the view that such a learning community would be able to make the real changes that a five-year project could not possibly effect.

Since each of these two assumptions was important in determining how we took action for learning, we briefly situate these assumptions in discourses of health promotion and capacity building. The first assumption was that cardiovascular disease prevention requires a population-based approach. There is a fundamental paradox at the core of understanding the determinants of heart health. On the one hand, individuals suffer from cardiovascular disease, and the choices made by individuals with regard to behaviours in the areas of smoking, nutrition, and exercise have a clear impact on their heart health. On the other hand, individuals' choices and behaviours are always structured by the social and material environments in which they live and over which they have limited influence. Differential mortality rates across social groups are only partially explainable by individual behaviours. The conceptual relationship between the agency of individual human beings and the constraints imposed upon them by social structures has been an enduring debate in social theory and in health promotion practice (Berger and Luckmann 1966; Bourdieu 1977; Smith 1990; Evans, Barer, and Marmor 1994; Feather 1994b; Feather and Labonte 1995; Raphael 2002, 2003). In contemplating heart health promotion activities, one must recognize that the determinants of heart health involve a complex interaction of individual behaviour and social structure. Labonte (Health Canada 1993, 9) has developed a useful model of the determinants of heart health (see Figure 2.1).

Within each category of risk identified in Figure 2.1, additional factors or conditions can be identified. For example, a more complete set of risk conditions would refer to the political economy of the agri-food industry, the sociology of urban planning and consumer culture, and the organization of labour processes, both paid and domestic, which fatigue people without stimulating their cardiovascular systems. The key point is that heart health promotion strategies cannot be reduced to a struggle against physiological or behavioural risk factors, when the determinants of heart health involve a complex interaction of such risk factors with social risk conditions and their psychosocial correlates.

Figure 2.1 implies a typology of strategic alternatives for combating cardiovascular disease (Health Canada 1993, 7). At the most structural level, social change and community development could be advanced to ameliorate the risk conditions experienced by disadvantaged populations. At the most individual level, medical or social-psychological interven-

Figure 2.1

Determinants of heart health

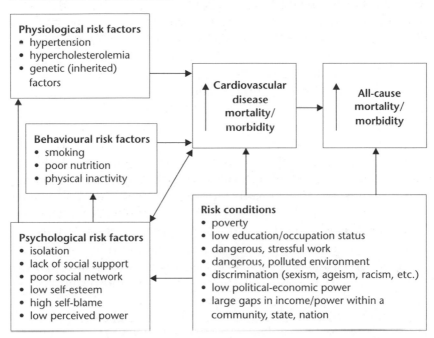

Source: Health Canada (1993). Reproduced with the permission of the Minister of Public Works and Government Services Canada, 2004.

tions could be implemented to treat people's physiological risk factors or change their behavioural risk factors.

Our approach to heart health promotion was a contextually specific one. We believed that there could be no a priori, abstract determination of a universally valid approach to promoting heart health. Different communities have different cultural, social, and political-economic characteristics, and a strategic assessment of such historical and contextual factors, not some abstract philosophical preference, should inform the approaches to heart health promotion used with each particular community. For us, building capacity for heart health promotion was therefore not a matter of disseminating particular programmatic interventions. Rather, it was a matter of nurturing, among communities of practitioners and leaders, the knowledge, skills, and commitment required to work with communities to explore the determinants of their populations' health, assess what could be done to influence those determinants, and take appropriate action.

Our conceptualization of health promotion and health promotion capacity was influenced by the existence of substantial literature produced by the early 1990s. A range of potential approaches to addressing the determinants of health had been examined by many authors, including Barnsley (1992); Bracht and Tsouros (1990); Butterfoss, Goodman, and Wandersman (1993); Downie, Fyfe, and Tannahill (1990); Epp (1986); Goodman and Steckler (1990); Green, Richard, and Potvin (1996); Israel et al. (1994); Jackson, Mitchell, and Wright (1989); Labonte (1987, 1993a, 1993b, 1993c, 1994); Rogers (1987); Shapiro, Cartwright, and Macdonald (1994); Wallack (1994); and the World Health Organization (1986). At the same time, the concept of capacity to engage in health promotion had been explored by a number of significant texts, including those by Bracht (1990); Elder et al. (1994); Ewles and Simnett (1992); Green and Kreuter (1991); Health and Welfare Canada (1992b); Kelleher (1996); Schwartz et al. (1993); and Tones and Tilford (1994). The concept of capacity continued, over the course of the BHPC project, to be a major focus of research and professional practice in health promotion (Casebeer, Scott, and Hannah [2000]; Chavis [1995]; Clark and McLeroy [1995]; Crisp, Swerissen, and Duckett [2000]; Elliot et al. [1998]; Freudenberg et al. [1995]; Goodman et al. [1998]; Hawe et al. [1997, 1998]; Kang [1995]; Kwan et al. [2003]; Mitchell and Sackney [2000]; Poole [1997]; and Smith, Littlejohns, and Thompson [2001]).

Our second key assumption had to do with the nature of capacity building, as dissemination. By the early 1990s, a substantial number of models of dissemination had been developed in the field of health promotion (see, for example, Basch et al. 1986; Monahan and Scheirer 1988; Orlandi et al. 1990; and Schwartz et al. 1993). However, our understanding of dissemination is rooted in Rogers's insightful review (1993) of the historical evolution of practices in agricultural extension and adult education. He argues that both disciplines evolved through three basic "generations of activity," characterized by fundamentally different understandings of processes of innovation, diffusion, and learning. While offered as a historical description of other fields, these three generations provide a conceptually attractive set of alternatives for thinking about dissemination and capacity building in the field of health promotion.

Figure 2.2 outlines a familiar, top-down approach to the diffusion of expertise. In this paradigm, knowledge is created through scientific research, and transferred to relatively passive target populations by the training and intervention of field workers. In terms of building health promotion capacity, this paradigm is reflected in the common practice of diffusing a "kit" of resources, which practitioners can then use in their practice.

Figure 2.2

Transfer of knowledge paradigm

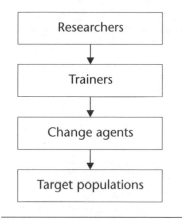

While many practitioners understand and appreciate the benefits of receiving knowledge (or other resources) from those possessing such knowledge, the transfer of knowledge paradigm is actually of limited utility for building capacity in complex areas such as health promotion. The transfer of knowledge paradigm does not allow the target populations to define what sort of knowledge they are to receive, or to ensure that what is disseminated matches their contextually specific needs and aspirations. Further, this paradigm exhibits a passive and disempowering understanding of members of the target population. It is an expert-driven paradigm that does little to nurture critical thinking skills on the part of target populations, and does not model the kinds of participatory approaches that are the hallmark of excellent health promotion practice.

Figure 2.3 outlines an alternative paradigm, whose point of departure consists of the needs of the target population rather than the scientific agenda of the researcher. In this second paradigm, the identification of problems, issues, and priorities emerges from needs assessment processes. Change agents and trainers act as informants and interpreters in the needs assessment processes. However, while the creation of new knowledge is responsive to the needs of target populations, the application and dissemination of that knowledge to the needs of the population is still quite directive. As in the first paradigm, the meeting needs paradigm presumes that target populations cannot meet their needs without sustained expert intervention. In terms of building health promotion capacity, this paradigm of dissemination is reflected in community

Figure 2.3

Meeting needs paradigm

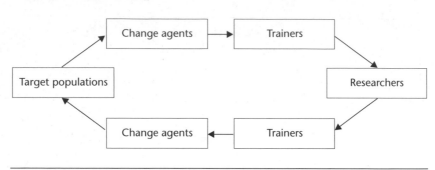

mobilization strategies that use conventional program planning cycles of needs assessment, implementation, and evaluation.

While the meeting needs paradigm provides a useful feedback loop to ensure that research outputs have some pertinence to the needs and aspirations of target populations, it still places those target populations in a state of dependency on knowledge generated elsewhere. Figure 2.4 outlines a model of the dissemination process that has a stronger affinity with community development approaches to health promotion. In this third paradigm, researchers and change agents recognize that target populations are actively engaged in dealing with issues and problems, and ultimately have responsibility for the resolution of those issues and problems. In this paradigm, the role of researchers and change agents is to share, in a reciprocal manner, knowledge and resources that will empower target populations to become even more effective and self-reliant.

In the BHPC project, we conceptualized our approach to capacity building as the development of interdependent learning communities. As discussed earlier in this chapter, the learners with whom we inter-

Figure 2.4

Developing independent learners paradigm

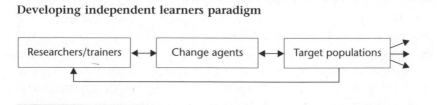

acted most centrally were health promotion practitioners employed by health districts across Saskatchewan.

Conclusion: From Discourse to Action

In this chapter, we set the stage for understanding what we did in the BHPC project, and what we learned from it. We provided a general background to our work by identifying some key elements of life in Saskatchewan in the late twentieth century. We then described changes to health policy, including the regionalization of health services administration, that characterized the province in the 1990s. In this context, we described how we worked, both at material and conceptual levels. We explained why we invested time, energy, and resources in building the capacity of health districts and health promotion practitioners to engage in population health promotion activities.

The next two chapters describe how we took action in order to build the capacity of individuals and organizations to promote health across Saskatchewan, and how we took action to better understand the process of capacity building. Chapters 5 through 7 then address, at the levels of individuals, organizations, and environments, what we learned about building capacity for health promotion work. The contextual and conceptual introduction presented in Chapter 2 should inform the reading of the rest of this book. That is, the manner in which we took action for learning and what we learned from that action were grounded in the context in which we worked, and were filtered through the conceptual frameworks with which we understood that work.

Part 2
Action for Learning

3
Understanding Health Promotion Capacity

Through the Building Health Promotion Capacity (BHPC) project, we took action for learning in two fundamental ways. First, we built our own knowledge. We designed a series of research activities to gain a better understanding of health promotion capacity and its development among individuals and organizations. Second, we facilitated the learning of others. We designed a series of interventions to enhance the knowledge, skills, and commitment of health promotion practitioners and leaders across Saskatchewan. These interventions were designed to help such practitioners and leaders to better understand, embrace, and implement population health promotion activities.

Although Chapters 3 and 4 present "research" and "intervention" as though they were distinct, we consistently strove to blend these two forms of action for learning in at least three ways. First, we followed a program planning cycle in which our continuing education interventions were based upon needs assessment research. These interventions were then evaluated, and evaluation results were used to plan future interventions. Second, we strove to make our research processes a learning opportunity for those who participated in our research. In most of the research instruments and procedures discussed in this chapter, we explicitly endeavoured to help our research participants reflect about their (or their organization's) health promotion capacity and what could be done to enhance that capacity. Third, we served as participant-observers in the interventions of our program. The interventions themselves were opportunities to gather qualitative data about the processes of learning that were taking place among participants, and about the health promotion capacity of those participants. Thus, while this chapter presents our research methods and the next chapter describes our interventions, the processes of research and intervention were interconnected.

Our research practices cannot be understood in isolation from our capacity-building interventions or from who we are as individuals and professionals. The past experiences of the BHPC team constituted a significant source of insight into issues surrounding capacity for health promotion in Saskatchewan, and structured the manner in which we endeavoured to learn more about such capacity. The staff members of BHPC had many years of experience as independent consultants and staff members with organizations such as the Prairie Region Health Promotion Research Centre, the Heart and Stroke Foundation of Saskatchewan, and the Saskatchewan Heart Health Program. Of the four faculty members with the BHPC research team, two were professors of Community Health and Epidemiology, one was a professor of Extension, and one was the province's Chief Medical Health Officer. At an informal level, our collective intuition, reflections, and conversations with colleagues contributed to our understanding of health promotion capacity and how it could be developed. More formally, BHPC team members had already participated in numerous research and continuing education initiatives involving health promotion practitioners and leaders across Saskatchewan.

This chapter outlines the research practices through which we took action to learn about the process of building health promotion capacity. We provide sufficient methodological detail with regard to those practices so that our readers will be able to understand how we formed our claims about health promotion capacity and its development.

Objectives and Methods

Our basic research objective was to build the scholarly and practical understanding of capacity and capacity building in health promotion. To accomplish this, we organized a five-year program of applied research that involved efforts to build health promotion capacity among individual practitioners and regional health districts in Saskatchewan, and efforts to examine and understand the process of capacity building. We understood capacity as being a characteristic of individual practitioners and of the organizations with which those practitioners worked. We conceptualized capacity as a set of knowledge, skills, commitment, and resources required by individuals and organizations to plan, implement, and evaluate effective health promotion activities. Capacity building was the process whereby such individuals and organizations became better able to undertake such activities. Capacity building was used as an alternative to the concept of dissemination, which can be understood as a planned, systematic process whereby new or existing knowledge, interventions, or practices are adopted, integrated, implemented, and maintained by a target population or populations. While we maintained the use of the term "capacity" throughout BHPC, we consistently used the term "capacity building" rather than "dissemination" in our work. This is largely due to the unfortunate association of "dissemination" with technology transfer models in which those who know (or have) disseminate information to those who do not know (or do not have). Our intention was to learn about capacity development alongside our research participants, and to respect the depth of knowledge that already existed among those participants.

Our interest in studying health promotion capacity and its development was stimulated by a pragmatic concern with population health in Saskatchewan and elsewhere. We assumed that health promotion capacity would enable practitioners and organizations to more effectively engage in health promotion action, and that such action would have a positive influence on the health status of people in Saskatchewan. Further, we assumed that supporting the continuing education and networking of practitioners and leaders would build their capacity to undertake, promote, and support health promotion work. Finally, we assumed that health promotion capacity and its development would be strongly influenced by environmental factors.

Given that our fundamental objective was to understand the processes through which capacity for health promotion work could be built among individuals and organizations, these assumptions were not translated into hypotheses to be tested through the gathering of evidence to reject the implicit null hypotheses. Rather, we used these assumptions to focus an exploratory and descriptive analysis of capacity-building processes. Our research methods were designed to advance the scholarly and practical understanding of capacity and how capacity is built, but were not intended to provide a statistically powerful set of tests to determine the extent to which capacity had been built.

To explore the process of capacity building among individual practitioners and health districts in Saskatchewan, we engaged in six distinct research methods. First, to establish the basic parameters of capacity and its development among health promotion practitioners and health districts, we conducted surveys. Second, to better understand the environment for health promotion in Saskatchewan, we conducted key informant interviews. Third, to explore health promotion capacity and capacity building in more detail, we conducted interviews and undertook modest case study research in two health districts. Fourth, to explore specific key issues related to health promotion capacity and its enhancement, we hosted think tanks. Fifth, to examine the contribution of our continuing education interventions to building capacity for health promotion work, we carefully evaluated the most significant of those interventions. Sixth, to capture the insights of our staff members as participant-observers, we gathered reflections from those staff members and held team retreats to share and synthesize our observations. To explain more fully how we went about taking action for learning about building health promotion capacity in Saskatchewan, the following sections describe these research methods in detail.

Surveys

To explore health promotion capacity among health promotion practitioners, we designed and implemented the Health Promotion Contact Profile. Between 1993 and 2002, each health district in Saskatchewan had a "Health Promotion Contact" (HPC). The HPCs played key roles in coordinating health promotion activities within their districts, and represented their districts to Saskatchewan Health on health promotion matters. To explore health promotion capacity among the thirty health districts in southern and central Saskatchewan, we designed and implemented the Health District Capacity Survey. The Health Promotion Contact Profile was sent to the HPCs, while the Health District Capacity Survey was sent to the chief executive officer of each district. A different version of each survey was sent three times: in autumn of 1998, in spring of 2000, and in winter of 2001-2. A fourth survey was initially planned but was not carried out because of the substantial reorganization of the health districts in 2002.

The development of our survey instruments involved the active participation of practitioners and other representatives of health districts whose capacity we were trying to understand and measure. This was important to us not only to enhance the validity of our subsequent data but also to model the type of participatory approach that we believe is integral to health promotion. From 1996 to 1998, we conducted literature reviews and other background work to conceptualize the capacity of individuals and organizations to engage in health promotion work. In May 1998 we hosted a think tank with provincial and national health promotion practitioners and researchers to review our conceptualization of capacity and to explore our ideas about measuring capacity. This think tank informed the creation of our two original survey instruments. From June to September 1998, we continued to consult with practitioners and organizational leaders across Saskatchewan to determine their views about how we had conceptualized capacity and to pretest the draft surveys through which we proposed to measure capacity. This consultation included correspondence and a formal session during the Health Promotion Contacts' provincial meeting in June 1998. Careful consultation with the subsequent respondents to the surveys was important to ensure a reasonably common understanding of the terms used in the surveys. It was also an effective means of encouraging a high response rate. In October and November 1998, the two surveys were distributed for completion. Twenty-seven of 30 (90 percent) Health Promotion Contact Profiles were returned, and 26 of 30 (87 percent) Health District Capacity Surveys were returned.

The 1998 HPC Profile explored respondents' knowledge of the determinants of health, skills in health promotion practice, and confidence with regard to the use of different health promotion strategies. The profile asked respondents to describe up to three health promotion initiatives in which they were currently engaged. Finally, the 1998 profile gathered information about respondents' socio-demographic characteristics and professional experiences, and asked the respondents to indicate what they would most need in order to strengthen their health promotion work.

The 1998 Health District Capacity Survey explored respondents' assessment of their health districts' organizational culture, commitment, processes, and practices with regard to health promotion. The survey asked respondents to identify the three most significant barriers to health promotion work in their districts, and to rate the importance of a range of factors that influence such work. Finally, the survey examined respondents' perceptions of their districts' current level of ability and engagement in health promotion activities, and asked respondents to indicate what they would most need in order to strengthen health promotion work in their districts.

Following the analysis of the 1998 surveys, we drew four conclusions about our survey research methodology. First, we realized that the survey instruments of 1998 were too long and placed a significant burden on their respondents. Second, we recognized that these survey instruments focused on the nature of capacity and its measurement, and did not adequately explore the dynamic process of capacity building. Third, we concluded that the survey instruments were able to provide some indication of the level of practitioners' and organizational leaders' knowledge and skill with regard to health promotion, but they did not effectively explore the elements of commitment and resources that we believed were also important components of capacity. Fourth, we realized that the largely closed-ended nature of the questions in the 1998 surveys prevented our respondents from explaining more fully the meaning of their experience with health promotion capacity and its development. These four conclusions led us to substantially revise the two survey instruments before using them a second time.

In our second round of surveys, administered in spring of 2000, the response rates were 26 of 30 (87 percent) for the HPC Profile and 27 of 30 (90 percent) for the Health District Capacity Survey. The second HPC Profile was substantially shorter and more open-ended than that of 1998. It explored respondents' intentional capacity-building activities and their impressions of changes to their capacity over the preceding year. It asked respondents to describe up to three incidents that had influenced the development of their health promotion capacity over the preceding year, and to rate the importance of a range of resources to their health promotion practice. Finally, the 2000 HPC Profile asked respondents to describe how their health promotion practices had changed over the preceding year, and to indicate what they would most like to do to enhance their future practices.

The 2000 Health District Capacity Survey explored respondents' assessments of their districts' health promotion capacity over the preceding year. It asked respondents to identify up to three intentional capacity-building efforts that their districts had made in the preceding year, and up to three incidents that had influenced the development of their districts' capacity over that time frame. Finally, the survey explored finances and partnerships as resources for health promotion work, and asked respondents what they would like to do to enhance their districts' health promotion capacity.

Between the second and third administrations of our survey instruments, a major transformation began in the health district system in Saskatchewan. Simply stated, the thirty health districts that had been our primary units of analysis were reorganized into twelve regional health authorities. This administrative reorganization obviously created a significant challenge to our original survey plans. Rather than being able to survey practitioners and leaders from thirty districts at four points in time over five years, we had to scramble to complete a third round of surveys before our units of analysis disappeared. The final HPC Profile and Health District Capacity Survey were designed as opportunities for respondents to reflect upon the evolution of their personal and organizational capacity for health promotion work, at a point in time at which the organizational context for that work was about to change significantly. Despite these challenging circumstances, the response rate among

HPCs was a remarkable 29 of 30 (97 percent). The response rate among respondents to the Health District Capacity Survey was understandably disappointing, at 19 of 30 (63 percent).

The 2001 HPC Profile was a two-stage process. The first stage was a written questionnaire that repeated key questions from the HPC Profiles of 1998 and 2000. The second stage was an in-depth telephone interview designed to increase our understanding of the capacity-building process. First, HPCs were asked to elaborate on their responses to the written profile. They explained their closed-ended responses and provided richer descriptions of specific areas in which they had experienced improvements in knowledge and skills, as well as changes in resources, practice, and overall health promotion capacity. Second, HPCs described the consequences or spin-offs of greater health promotion capacity. Third, HPCs created a personal timeline of the past year and described two events or circumstances that had been particularly influential in shaping their practice. For each event, the HPCs described what happened, how they reacted to the event, what key insights or learnings they took away from the event, and what implications stemmed from the event. Fourth, HPCs commented on further actions they might take to improve their individual health promotion capacity.

The interview guide was modified for some respondents. Ten HPCs went beyond the one-year time frame to provide a narrative of career experience. This permitted an exploration of milestones that had shaped the development of the practitioners' capacity over the course of a career. Several HPCs who were involved in building organizational capacity within their districts were asked to highlight steps, challenges, and accomplishments in that process. This version of the interview helped us to better understand the interaction between individual and organizational capacity.

Our final Health District Capacity Survey was administered in February 2002. The 2002 survey repeated key questions from the two earlier surveys. Like the final HPC Profile, the 2002 Health District Capacity Survey had a second, qualitative follow-up stage. Rather than interview each CEO, however, we deliberately sampled three health districts (one urban and two rural) for a facilitated "organizational time line" exercise. This time line exercise was designed to build our understanding of how factors and events interacted and unfolded in health districts to shape health promotion capacity. District representatives were invited to participate in a retreat to explore critical events and steps in the development of health promotion in their districts. Critical events were identified through a visioning exercise, where participants reflected on the evolution of health promotion in their district since its inception in 1992. Before the retreat, a time line was drawn on a long sheet of paper, with years marked from 1992 to 2002. Along the time line, signposts were drawn and significant provincial and national events were posted. Participants were invited to add to the time line by noting the events they had remembered through the visioning. Events specific to their districts went on the time line; other events that were significant personally went on a flip chart sheet marked "self"; and other provincial events not already on the time line went on a sheet marked "provincial." Following a review of the events, participants were asked to vote on the three events on the district timeline that they felt were most critical in their districts with respect to health promotion. For each of the three events, participants then elaborated on what had happened, how they as a district had reacted to the event, what the district had learned from the event, and decisions made in response to the event. As a summary of the process, participants were asked about final reflections on their time line, the health promotion legacy of their districts, and implications for further health promotion capacity development within their new regional health authority.

In summary, the six surveys we undertook during the BHPC project were important sources of data about the health promotion capacity of practitioners and health districts in Saskatchewan, and about how such capacity changed over time. Our survey instruments were largely quantitative at first, but eventually involved qualitative interviews and focus group processes.

Key Informant Interviews
To better understand the environment for health promotion in Saskatchewan, we conducted key informant interviews with individuals believed to have credible insight into provincial and national contexts. We conducted two rounds of ten key informant interviews; the first began in January 1999 and the second in January 2000. There was some overlap in respondents in the two rounds. Respondents included senior officials with Saskatchewan Health as well as practitioners and managers in community and public agencies other than health districts. Each interview:

• explored the respondent's understanding of population health and population health promotion

- invited the respondent's assessment of the health promotion capacity of his or her own organization as well as that of health districts and the province as a whole
- invited the respondent to identify federal and provincial policies or funding changes affecting health promotion programs or activities, and any other relevant and significant national or international trends that may have affected the provincial health promotion scene
- inquired about social, economic, political, or cultural changes influencing health promotion in the province
- asked about shifts in practice guidelines for clinicians or others that were or could have been influencing health promotion actions
- asked about the impact of any continuing education events, other than those of BHPC, on health promotion capacity in the province
- inquired about awareness of the BHPC project and its impact on the health promotion scene
- requested identification of actions or factors influencing public acceptance of health promotion
- asked for the identification of one or two developments (policies, programs, events, etc.) with significant impact on the health of the people of the province

The interviews were conducted by telephone, tape-recorded, and transcribed. The key informant interviews were an excellent source of data regarding the environment for health promotion in Saskatchewan.

Case Studies
To explore health promotion capacity and capacity building in more detail than was possible through survey research, we conducted interviews and undertook modest participant-observation research in two health districts. The case study districts were selected in a two-stage process. In the first stage, we identified a number of districts with widely differing sizes and existing levels of health promotion activity. In the second stage, we invited districts to volunteer. Out of the fourteen districts that volunteered, we signed formal agreements with two. Part of the agreement was that we would not reveal the identity of the case study districts to anyone outside each specific district, not even to the other case study district.

With mutual agreement as to timing, we visited these districts to observe board and committee meetings, to conduct face-to-face interviews with key staff members, and to meet with district managers to discuss events and developments in the districts. Both districts provided written documentation of their plans, programs, and progress. As anticipated, the two districts continued to vary in their capacity and health promotion initiatives. They also varied in their capacity to accommodate our data collection efforts. At times, events in a district would place sufficient demands on the local management team to preclude our taking up their time with interviews. In those circumstances, we relied on observation of meetings and informal discussions with management. One of the districts agreed to participate in the organizational time line process described above; the other did not because of disruptions related to the restructuring of the districts into regional health authorities.

In addition to our work with the case study districts, we had initially planned to collect documents from a number of "case monitoring" districts. We recruited ten districts to send us documents such as annual reports, annual health plans, strategic plans, newsletters, media releases, and minutes of health promotion committees. This relatively unobtrusive research method was not pursued past the first year of BHPC. We did not have the resources to analyze adequately the content of the documents we received, and the documents themselves turned out to be of such diversity that they were too difficult to analyze for indications of health promotion capacity and its evolution over time.

Think Tanks

To explore specific issues related to health promotion capacity and its enhancement, we held think tanks with selected participants. During the BHPC project, we hosted three think tank meetings that, in methodological terms, shared certain characteristics of focus groups. In May 1998 we hosted a two-stage think tank of health promotion practitioners and researchers to review our preliminary conceptualization of capacity building and to explore our ideas about measuring capacity. The first stage was a one-day meeting of exemplary health promotion practitioners from around Saskatchewan. Eight invited practitioners from government, urban and rural health districts, and the not-for-profit sector gathered to discuss the practice realities of health promotion in Saskatchewan health districts, identify elements of health promotion capacity, and discuss implications for BHPC strategic planning. This day elicited a Saskatchewan vision of a capacity-rich environment within which health promotion could flourish. It also helped identify the assets, limitations, and qualities of an individual with high capacity for health promotion work. The second stage of the think tank brought together seven experienced researchers from across Canada for one and a half days. This stage of the process was designed to draw on the experiences of others engaged in health promotion and capacity-building research in order to build on our conceptualization of health promotion capacity.

Whereas our first think tank was dedicated to exploring the conceptualization and measurement of health promotion capacity, our second think tank explored the context of health promotion work in Saskatchewan and assessed the implications of that context for the design of interventions to build capacity for health promotion. Our second think tank was held in June 1999 and involved nine participants in addition to BHPC staff. Seven represented different health districts and two represented Saskatchewan Health. The think tank explored the following questions:

- What would health districts look like if they had the highest possible health promotion capacity?
- What are the challenges and opportunities in building health promotion capacity in the health districts?
- What are the current and potential roles of think tank participants in building health promotion capacity?
- Who are the key players influencing health promotion capacity in the health districts?
- How can BHPC contribute to the enhancement of health promotion capacity in the health districts?

Our third think tank, held in October 2000, engaged fourteen leaders and scholars from across Saskatchewan in a dialogue with BHPC staff and researchers about the context and potential opportunities for health promotion in the province. Participants included leaders with Saskatchewan Health, Health Canada, the health districts, the Saskatchewan Association of Health Organizations, the Health Services Utilization and Research Commission, the Human Services Integration Forum, and the Saskatchewan Population Health and Evaluation Research Unit. The think tank explored the context of the present health care system and the opportunities and potential solutions for strengthening the role of health promotion in that system and beyond. The think tank then examined implications of this exploration for the intervention and research work of the BHPC project.

Evaluation Research
To examine the contribution of our continuing education interventions

to building capacity for health promotion work, we carefully evaluated the process and impact of the most significant of those interventions. The overall framework for this evaluation research was provided by Kirkpatrick's four levels (1994) of satisfaction, learning, behaviour change, and impact:

- *Satisfaction.* How satisfied were the participants with the educational experience that was provided?
- *Learning.* What (if any) new knowledge, skills, or attitudes did participants learn as a result of the intervention?
- *Behaviour change.* Did learning accomplished through the intervention result in changes to the professional practices of the participants?
- *Impact.* Did the participants' changed practices result in an impact on organizations or communities?

To varying degrees, we assembled evidence for each of these four levels in an attempt to understand and document our continuing education intervention. The rigour with which we evaluated our interventions varied with the investment that was made in those interventions, and with our degree of control over the evaluation process. At one end of the continuum, major interventions such as the health promotion summer schools were evaluated carefully through on-site surveys and follow-up interviews. At the other end of the continuum, short presentations made to external conferences were not evaluated beyond the superficial satisfaction surveys conducted by the organizers of those conferences.

Participant Observation
To capture the insights of our staff members as participant-observers engaged in a complex set of research and intervention activities, we gathered "reflection notes" from staff and held team retreats to share and synthesize our observations. Following each intervention, members of the team recorded their observations and thoughts regarding both the effectiveness of methods used and the response of the participants. We also recorded notes on significant informal conversations we had with event participants, and on what we were learning about capacity through the specific event. Such reflections were brought to monthly staff meetings. Minutes of those meetings were recorded, including reflections, debate, and discussion about capacity development. Once or twice per year, full BHPC meetings created opportunities for staff and investigators to work together to understand what was being learned. On these occasions, we engaged in small-group processes to

compile insights from direct observation as well as the analysis of other data sources.

Claims to Knowledge and the Presentation of Evidence

While Chapters 3 and 4 indicate how we took action for learning, Chapters 5, 6, and 7 describe the learning that took place from that action. In those three chapters, we make a series of claims about the nature of health promotion capacity and how it develops. These claims are rooted in the intervention and research practices described in this and the next chapter. At this point, we outline the epistemological assumptions that underpin our claims to knowledge, and then describe the concrete practices of analysis through which we developed those claims.

To understand the manner in which we provide evidence for our claims to knowledge, it is necessary to be aware of the debate between research traditions that we have elsewhere contrasted as "positivism" and "interpretive humanism" (McLean 1999). Positivism, in many ways the orthodox approach to social science, views social life as resembling the natural world, and suggests that social scientific inquiry should resemble the natural sciences. Interpretive humanism views social life as resembling a work of art or a literary text, and suggests that social scientific inquiry must strive to understand the thoughts and feelings of the actors who create that world. Although our work contains elements of the positivist research tradition, we are making claims to knowledge largely from an interpretive humanist perspective.

The positivist and interpretive humanist research traditions have fundamentally different assumptions about the manner through which knowledge about the social world may be created and validated. The positivist tradition argues that the natural sciences provide a model for knowing social life. Social phenomena such as "capacity" and "capacity building," which do not seem to be directly accessible through empirical observation, can be operationalized, observed, and measured through scientific procedures such as experiments, attitudinal scales, and social surveys. The adequacy of knowledge derived from such methods is determined by other scientists' replication of empirical observations, and by the construction and testing of theories that explain such empirical observations and that can be falsified through repeated observations.

In contrast, the interpretive humanist tradition rejects empirical observation as a sufficient foundation from which to generate knowledge about the social world. Since the social world does not exist outside its actors' inter-subjective interpretations of that world, interpretive humanist researchers use a hermeneutic approach to understanding the meaning of people's actions. Rather than seeking inspiration in the natural sciences, the model for social scientific research is found in the humanities' methods for interpreting written texts or artistic creations. Interpretive humanists suggest that valid knowledge of the social world is derived from the construction of interpretive understandings of the meaning of social interaction for its participants. The adequacy of such knowledge is determined by the degree to which it makes sense both to the participants directly involved in the social action being interpreted and to a community of scholars engaged in the interpretation of similar actions.

In more concrete terms, how did we actually validate the claims to knowledge that we make in this book? In short, we validated our claims through sustained engagement with our research participants. We came to understand capacity and capacity building through interacting with the people and organizations whose capacity formed the object of our research. As discussed in this and the next chapter, our continuing education and research practices were developed through ongoing consultation with the "learners" and "research subjects" of those practices. Our claims to knowledge about capacity and its development were initially made in the form of curricula and research instruments. Throughout the process of engaging in research and continuing education about health promotion capacity, we talked with the participants of our research about the ideas we had generated. These discussions led us to revise our continuing education and research practices, and such revised practices led to changes in our claims to knowledge about capacity and its development. The cyclical engagement of our research participants in reflection on claims to knowledge about capacity is the source of the strongest evidence we can provide with regard to those claims. In essence, we know that our claims to knowledge are valid because they make sense to those whose capacity was the focus of our claims. Our research participants have found great insight and value in our claims to knowledge, and have, over a significant period of sustained contact, helped us to refine those claims.

In addition to the process of verifying the consensus of our research participants, triangulation and inter-subjective dialogue have been important means of validating our claims to knowledge. Triangulation was made possible by the multiple forms of action that we took to learn about health promotion capacity. The six categories of research methods outlined in this chapter, and the interventions described in the next chapter, gave us many ways of looking at capacity and its development.

Inter-subjective dialogue was the cornerstone of our data analysis processes. Each of our major claims to knowledge was developed by teams of BHPC staff members reviewing various data sources and comparing their interpretations of those sources. While such inter-subjective dialogue took place over the course of BHPC, it was intensively practised during two periods in which we more or less stopped gathering data and conducting continuing education. These periods were from October 2000 through June 2001 and from January through June 2003.

In order to present our learning from action in the most coherent and compelling manner, Chapters 5 through 7 do not include substantial direct evidence for the claims that we have made. To do so would have meant increasing the length of each chapter and diluting our basic argument about capacity with direct citations from our research participants. Ultimately, it is what we have learned that is of primary interest and importance to readers of this book; the evidence to support our claims about what we have learned reflects the methods described in this chapter but is not presented in subsequent chapters.

Conclusion

In this chapter, we have described the methods by which we took action for learning about the evolution of capacity to engage in health promotion work in Saskatchewan. Besides providing details of our various research methods, this chapter has indicated that our overall approach to research changed over time. First, our focus shifted from trying to understand the health promotion capacity of individuals and organizations to trying to understand the processes through which the health promotion capacity of individuals and organizations changes over time. Second, our research activities evolved from relatively more quantitative to relatively more qualitative over time. While the measurement of capacity is both a quantitative and qualitative challenge, the understanding of how capacity changes is fundamentally qualitative: it requires research methods that capture historical and biographical narratives and engage the creators of those narratives in critical dialogue about how and why changes have taken place. Third, the external environment had a decisive impact on our ability to take action for learning to understand health promotion capacity in Saskatchewan. The reorganization of the health district system in the province played havoc with our original research intentions. Some of our units of analysis essentially disappeared, while others were so preoccupied with the consequences of this reorganization that their time and energy for engaging in research were substantially diminished.

The theme of a complex and unpredictable environment constraining rational planning and action is one that will be repeated in our later chapters on learning from action. Just as our research methods were challenged by real-world events beyond our control, so the development of health promotion capacity by individuals and organizations was fundamentally shaped by environmental factors beyond the control of those individuals and organizations.

4
Building Health Promotion Capacity

This chapter describes how we facilitated the learning of others. We delivered an annual summer school on health promotion. We offered regional and provincial continuing education events concerning a range of health promotion topics. We created and facilitated an Internet listserv to enhance peer networking in the field of health promotion. We nurtured a strong working relationship with the Health Promotion Contacts (HPCs) employed by each of the health districts in Saskatchewan. We provided information about, and advocated for a commitment to, health promotion among health district leaders and senior managers. Finally, we worked to change the health promotion environment in Saskatchewan by providing a range of consulting services, supporting existing networks, and engaging in advocacy with the provincial department of health.

Through these forms of intervention, we acted to build capacity for health promotion in Saskatchewan. The interventions also enabled us to learn about the process of capacity building among individuals and organizations. We became active participants rather than detached observers in the complex changes that took place among health promotion practitioners and health districts over the course of our research. These interventions provided privileged insights into the dynamics of the capacity-building process.

This chapter provides substantial detail about the action for learning that we organized in order to build capacity for health promotion across Saskatchewan. Some readers may find that this level of detail is unnecessary, and simply skim this chapter in order to get more quickly to the lessons we learned from this action; other readers will appreciate knowing the details. To understand what we learned about health promotion capacity, it is important to know what we did to develop such capacity.

Health Promotion Summer Schools

Our major strategy for building health promotion capacity in Saskatchewan was to provide continuing education and networking opportunities to people involved with health promotion work. Organizing and delivering four health promotion summer schools was a cornerstone of this strategy. The Prairie Region Health Promotion Research Centre (PRHPRC) initiated Saskatchewan's health promotion summer schools in 1997, the year before the Building Health Promotion Capacity project began. From 1998 through 2003, the centre sponsored four summer schools, relying heavily on BHPC staff to design and implement learning plans in cooperation with other partnering organizations. The dates and themes of the summer schools were:

- 17-22 August 1998, Planning and Evaluating Population Health Promotion
- 15-20 August 1999, Moving from Principles to Practice in Population Health Promotion
- 14-18 August 2000, Working with Community: An Intersectoral Health Promotion Summer School
- 19-23 August 2002, Working for Change in the Community and in Organizations

Table 4.1 summarizes the attendance at these summer schools.

As indicated by their titles, each summer school had a distinct focus. In 1998, we focused on building the capacity of participants to effectively plan and evaluate health promotion activities. Specifically, we wanted to help participants become more effective at: (1) analyzing qualitative and quantitative data, (2) using information for planning, (3) planning for population health and acting on health determinants, (4) evaluating health promotion and community development, and (5) assessing evaluation reports.

Table 4.1

Attendance at health promotion summer schools, 1998-2002

	1998	1999	2000	2002
Registering as students	189	173	153	281
Faculty and staff	36	38	36	32
Total attendance	225	211	189	313

In 1999, the focus was on enabling health promotion practitioners to move from an understanding of the principles of health promotion to an ability to effectively undertake health promotion efforts. Each of the five days of the 1999 summer school was organized around a fundamental learning challenge for health promotion practitioners. The five challenges were: (1) mapping the causal linkages between the determinants of health and specific health outcomes, (2) grounding health promotion practice in values and principles, (3) choosing appropriate foci and strategies for health promotion action, (4) evaluating and reflecting critically on health promotion efforts; and (5) bringing learning from summer school back to an organizational context in order to make an impact on health promotion efforts. Our 1999 summer school was recognized with an award for program excellence from the Canadian Association for University Continuing Education.

In 2000, the overall purpose of the summer school was to provide an opportunity for personal and professional development in an intersectoral environment that would enable participants to learn and practise skills for working with communities. The learning content of summer school 2000 focused on: (1) key concepts of working intersectorally; (2) the program planning cycle; (3) facilitation skills, consensus building, and working in groups; (4) learning intersectorally; and (5) creating supportive learning environments to sustain action.

We did not host a summer school in 2001. At that time, BHPC staff members were heavily engaged in a mid-program data analysis process. They were also playing key roles in planning the annual meeting of the Canadian Public Health Association to be held in Saskatoon that fall, and the Build Better Tomorrows conference on diabetes prevention, scheduled for February 2002. In 2002, summer school returned, and addressed the theme of working for change in communities and organizations. The learning content included: (1) recognizing human-centred development as the goal of change, (2) understanding theories and processes of change in communities and organizations, (3) managing conflict and resistance to change, (4) building and maintaining relationships for change, and (5) evaluating and celebrating change.

While the summer schools addressed various themes, they shared four key elements. First, each summer school was intended to address a major capacity-building need of health promotion practitioners across Saskatchewan and beyond. The specific themes were based upon BHPC research processes and consultations with key stakeholders and selected practitioners. The fundamental purpose of the summer schools was to enhance health promotion action by building the knowledge, skills, and networks of practitioners. Most participants in the summer schools were from Saskatchewan, and most worked in health and other human services sectors. Each year, however, some participants came from other provinces and countries, and an increasing number of participants came from fields other than health.

Second, each summer school was organized with the participation of a significant number of partnering agencies:

- Saskatchewan Health (Population Health Branch)
- Health Canada (Health Promotion and Programs Branch, Health Protection Branch, Population and Public Health Branch)
- University of Saskatchewan (Department of Community Health and Epidemiology)
- Saskatchewan Human Services Integration Forum
- Saskatchewan Association of Health Organizations
- Saskatchewan Public Health Association
- Saskatoon Tribal Council
- Métis Nation of Saskatchewan
- Federation of Saskatchewan Indian Nations
- Saskatchewan Council for Community Development

These agencies provided several forms of assistance to the summer schools. Some of them, especially Saskatchewan Health and Health Canada, provided funding support in the form of grants or student bursaries. All of them worked on advisory committees (helping to shape the learning agenda and process) and helped to publicize the summer schools through their networks.

Third, the summer schools shared a commitment to innovative and effective pedagogical strategies. The 1998 summer school had a relatively conventional format, consisting largely of plenary and concurrent sessions in which participants listened to speakers and then had an opportunity to pose questions to those speakers. The next three summer schools adopted a more sophisticated approach to adult learning. Their format was revamped to better reflect effective adult education methods and to help participants better translate new knowledge and skills into practice. Participants in the last three summer schools spent about half their time in plenary sessions and half their time working in small, facilitated learning groups that stayed together over the course of the week. In 1999, these learning groups were organized into thirteen thematic areas ranging from "tobacco control" and "heart health promotion" to "reducing inequalities" and "sustainable ecosystems and communities." In 2000, participants were organized into ten regional working groups based on the Regional Intersectoral Committee boundaries in Saskatchewan, to foster subsequent networking and help people learn to work together. In 2002, the small groups were organized according to participants' focus on change in communities or change in organizations, and the participants' geographic settings (urban, rural, northern, or international).

In all three years, the small-group structure provided the following pedagogical benefits:

- It encouraged personal reflection and interpersonal discussion of ideas presented by plenary speakers.
- It enabled participants to orient their learning to issues and concerns of importance to them.
- It provided the opportunity to immediately apply new knowledge and skills in a supportive learning environment.
- It enabled participants to share their own experiences and make such experiences part of the learning process in their small group.
- It created a learning environment that promoted consistent attendance over the course of the week.
- It provided opportunities for building deeper personal bonds and networks between participants.
- It added flexibility to the conventional teaching and learning strategies of presentations and demonstrations (the small groups enabled participatory methods such as discussion, role playing, and collaborative case study analysis).
- It created a balance between theory (as presented during plenary sessions) and practice (as discussed and analyzed in small groups).

Fourth, the summer schools were resource-intensive. They required a tremendous amount of staff and faculty time to plan and implement. They involved excellent speakers and resource people. In addition to invited speakers, the three most recent summer schools engaged between ten and nineteen facilitators to work with the learning groups over the course of the week. A learning guide was developed to help ensure consistency between learning groups, and facilitators were given careful orientation to their roles. The facilitators met regularly throughout the week to check notes, compare progress, and make revisions to the planned small-group processes. The facilitators also provided feedback to the summer school planners with regard to the learning design. Such feedback was used as part of the evaluation process to improve the learning design for subsequent summer schools.

Besides the human resources involved in planning, teaching, and facilitating the summer schools, these continuing education events involved investment in the development and distribution of educational materials. Each participant received a substantial binder of resource materials pertinent to the theme of the summer school. In addition, a "bookstore" of carefully selected materials was assembled and made available to participants (for purchase) throughout each summer school. The immediate outcome of our investment of human and financial resources was consistently positive evaluation of the summer schools. The more significant outcome was a contribution to building capacity for health promotion across Saskatchewan.

The four summer schools were consistently evaluated through an onsite evaluation form, which asked participants to indicate their satisfaction with various sessions and aspects of the summer schools, and to self-assess their learning by indicating how well various objectives had been met. For the 1999 summer school, more intensive evaluation research was conducted through the completion of a master's thesis (Berkowitz 2000). This research involved follow-up questionnaires and interviews focusing on the changes to practitioners' health promotion practices as a result of their participation in the summer school. To summarize, participant satisfaction and self-assessed learning were consistently high. Participants rated the events highly, and were able to identify concrete and important lessons learned from participation in those events. We also know that some participants changed their professional practices as a result of what they learned at the summer schools. However, our systematic evidence regarding such behavioural change is limited to the 1999 summer school, and we also know that a range of organizational and environmental barriers hindered many participants from consistently applying what they learned.

The health promotion summer schools were a major continuing education intervention through which we endeavoured to make an impact on the knowledge, skills, and commitment of practitioners and leaders in health promotion across Saskatchewan. The summer schools were strategically designed in response to our perceptions of the most significant needs and aspirations of the practitioners and leaders we served. The teaching and learning processes evolved over time, as we became increasingly adept at using innovative and effective adult education methods. Evaluation results indicate that the summer schools had a substantial impact on the development of health promotion capacity among many individuals across Saskatchewan and beyond.

Provincial and Regional Continuing Education Events

In addition to the summer schools, BHPC offered, independently or in partnership with other organizations, eleven provincial or regional continuing education events between 1998 and 2002. Some were organized in response to requests from particular groups or to opportunities presented by the activities of other organizations; others were organized by BHPC as strategic interventions with groups that we identified as important to our overall concern with building health promotion capacity across Saskatchewan.

Table 4.2 provides the dates, titles, and numbers of participants of the provincial and regional continuing education events in which BHPC served as a primary organizer or partner.

The events listed in Table 4.2 fall into three basic categories: (1) five workshops for provincial audiences within specific professional categories, (2) four workshops for regional groupings of health districts, and (3) two large provincial events.

Workshops for Professional Groups

We organized five workshops for public health inspectors, public health nurses, and public health nutritionists across the province. In each case, BHPC staff worked with representatives of the target audience to assess their most pertinent learning needs and to design educational workshops to address those needs. We delivered two workshops to public health inspectors across the province, with the overall goal of building their capacity to contribute to population health promotion activities. The first, full-day workshop was delivered to twenty public health inspectors (from ten health districts) on 8 December 1998 in Regina. Its objectives were to enable public health inspectors to: (1) increase their understanding of basic health promotion concepts; (2) apply *A Population Health Promotion Framework for Saskatchewan Health Districts* to the practice of public health inspection; (3) identify factors that enable or impede health promotion activities in their work, and outline strategies to address these factors; and (4) develop public health inspection examples of health promotion practice to share with colleagues. The workshop included presentations, large-group discussions, and small-group activities.

Table 4.2

BHPC provincial and regional continuing education events

Date	Attendees	Event and location
8 December 1998	20	Public Health Inspectors Workshop: Integrating Health Promotion (Regina)
28 January 1999	14	Public Health Nurse Managers Workshop (Regina)
18 March 1999	14	Senior Public Health Inspectors Workshop: Integrating Health Promotion (Regina)
9 September 1999	52	Tri-District Health Promotion Workshop: Strengthening Health Promotion Practice (Melfort)
30 September 1999	>600	Michael Quinn Patton Telecast: Evaluating Intersectoral Programs: Meeting the Challenges (province-wide)
15 November 1999	21	Battlefords Service Area Health Promotion Workshop: Principles of Empowering Practice (North Battleford)
28 January 2000	36	Southeast Service Area Health Promotion Workshop: Strengthening Health Promotion Practice (Weyburn)
12-14 February 2002	314	Build Better Tomorrows Conference: Work Together on the Determinants of Health (Saskatoon)
30 April 2002	33	Southwest Service Area Health Promotion Workshop (Swift Current)
25 September 2002	17	Public Health Nutritionists Workshop: Strengthening Health Promotion Practice in Nutrition Programs (Saskatoon)
28 November 2002	14	Public Health Nurse Managers Workshop (Saskatoon)

As a follow-up to our work with the public health inspectors, we delivered a two-hour workshop with senior public health inspectors on 18 March 1999. Senior public health inspectors have supervisory responsibility for a group of public health inspectors, and therefore fill management roles in program planning, delivery, and evaluation. Twelve senior public health inspectors and two representatives of Saskatchewan Health took part. The workshop objectives were to enable senior public health inspectors to: (1) understand how the determinants of health influence the work of enforcing public health regulations, (2) learn the basic concepts of the population health promotion approach, and (3) discuss the challenges and benefits of adopting a population health promotion approach in public health inspection work. The workshop involved presentations and group discussion of the challenges and benefits of adopting a population health promotion approach in public health inspection work.

On 28 January 1999, we delivered a half-day workshop to twelve public health nurse managers with health districts across Saskatchewan and two provincial consultants from Saskatchewan Health. The workshop was designed to enable the managers to: (1) review the main ideas in *A Population Health Promotion Framework for Saskatchewan Health Districts,* (2) work though examples of meeting health challenges using critical analysis skills and the *Framework,* and (3) discuss the implications of the *Framework* for public health nursing practice. The workshop included presentations and a small-group exercise.

On 28 November 2002, we delivered a second half-day workshop to the public health nurse managers from across Saskatchewan. A dozen participants from the new regional health authorities took part, along with two employees of Saskatchewan Health. The objectives of the workshop were to: (1) increase understanding of health promotion capacity, (2) present options and strategies for building health promotion capacity, (3) facilitate the application of theory to participants' own practices, (4) contribute to the process of learning together as peers, and (5) identify next steps in building health promotion capacity. The workshop involved both presentations and group discussions.

On 25 September 2002, we delivered a one-day workshop for seventeen public health nutritionists from across Saskatchewan. The goal of the workshop was to strengthen their capacity to plan and evaluate public health nutrition and health promotion programs. Through participation in the workshop, participants were expected to be able to: (1) distinguish between health education, health promotion, population health promotion, and the three primary approaches to health promotion; (2) understand the elements of a program logic model; and (3) identify how program logic models can be used to support effective program planning and evaluation strategies. The workshop involved plenary presentations and the use of facilitated learning groups to develop program logic models related to interventions with populations in early childhood, later childhood, and adulthood.

Each of the five workshops for professional groups in the province was carefully planned and delivered. However, we did not evaluate these events beyond satisfaction and learning self-assessment surveys conducted at the end of each workshop. From these surveys, we know that most participants were reasonably satisfied with their learning experiences, and most believed they had learned something that they could apply to their professional practices. We did not invest further resources in evaluation because of the relatively modest time frame of each workshop.

Regional Workshops with Health District Personnel

We organized four workshops for multidisciplinary audiences working with regional groupings of health districts. Our first regional workshop was held on 9 September 1999 in Melfort, and involved 52 participants from Pasquai Health District (15), North Central Health District (22), and North East Health District (15). The goal of this one-day event was to strengthen health promotion practice by providing practitioners with opportunities to increase their understanding of basic health promotion concepts, assess their own practice against the principles of empowering practice, and identify opportunities to work cooperatively to strengthen health promotion. The title of the workshop was "Strengthening Health Promotion Practice," and its objectives were to enable participants to: (1) define and contrast health protection, health promotion, and the treatment and rehabilitation of illness; (2) understand the principles of empowering practice; (3) demonstrate how existing activities could be changed using the health promotion concept of empowering practice; (4) identify when implicit health promotion opportunities arise during regular professional activities; (5) identify explicit health promotion opportunities within health district strategic plans; and (6) meet colleagues from other health districts.

These objectives were pursued through a plenary presentation and small-group discussion and problem-solving sessions.

Our second regional workshop was held on 15 November 1999 in North Battleford, and involved ten participants from Battlefords Health District, four from Northwest Health District, three from Lloydminster Health District, two from Twin Rivers Health District, and one person with responsibilities across the service area. The workshop was designed to strengthen health promotion capacity by giving participants an opportunity to: (1) know how to use a program logic model in health promotion planning and evaluation, (2) strengthen skills in assessing health promotion activities against health promotion principles and values, (3) know what steps can be taken to strengthen health promotion practice at individual and organizational levels, and (4) strengthen connections between public health staff in the service area. These objectives were pursued through plenary presentations and small-group discussion and problem-solving sessions.

Our third regional workshop was held on 28 January 2000 in Weyburn, and involved 30 participants from Moose Mountain Health District (7), South Central Health District (12), and South East Health District (11), and 3 participants whose responsibilities covered two or more districts. The title of the workshop was "Strengthening Health Promotion Practice," and its objectives and methods were the same as those of the workshop held in North Battleford.

Our fourth regional workshop was held on 30 April 2002 in Swift Current, and involved 33 participants. Of the participants, 29 were employed by four health districts: Rolling Hills (16), Midwest (4), Southwest (6), and Swift Current (3). The rest were employed by educational institutions or the Regional Intersectoral Committee. Through their participation in the workshop, participants were expected to be able to: (1) define the eight key ideas of population health promotion, (2) describe their current practice strengths and challenges in relation to population health promotion, (3) identify future opportunities for population health promotion, and (4) know the elements of a program logic model and how it can be used to create effective health promotion program plans and evaluation strategies.

Our teaching and learning strategies for this event involved plenary presentations concerning the key ideas in population health promotion and the use of program logic models, as well as two facilitated learning group activities. The first activity asked participants to work in district groups to discuss the realities and challenges of putting population health promotion into action. The second activity asked participants to create a program logic model around one of five topics: early childhood development, youth, seniors, farm safety, or mental health.

Our regional events represented a substantial investment on our part and on the part of participating health districts. Before each workshop, BHPC staff interviewed a sample of participants to assess their health promotion practice strengths and learning needs. Workshops were planned in collaboration with regional steering committees. Each workshop was guided by a learning design that specified objectives, content, and processes. Given the substantial investment in these workshops, and given the fact that the participants in those events were central to our overall capacity-building efforts, we evaluated the regional workshops rather closely. We conducted on-site surveys of participant satisfaction and self-assessed learning, and we conducted follow-up interviews, from four to six months following each event, to examine behavioural change with a sample of participants from each event.

Complete results of our evaluation of these regional workshops are available in a series of reports (Saskatchewan Heart Health Program 1999a, 1999b, 2001, 2002a). Participant satisfaction with the workshops was good, but not as high as with the summer schools. Most participants believed they made considerable progress toward the learning objectives of the workshops, and many were able to identify specific insights about health promotion that they had gained from the workshops. Finally, most respondents to the follow-up interviews reported that changes to professional practices had taken place as a result of the workshops.

Provincial Events

Besides BHPC workshops, we partnered to deliver two large provincial events designed to address key health promotion learning needs in Saskatchewan. The first was a province-wide telecast, *Evaluating Intersectoral Programs: Meeting the Challenges,* held on 30 September 1999. Saskatchewan Health was the lead agency; its partners were BHPC, Health Canada, the Prairie Region Health Promotion Research Centre, and the Government of Saskatchewan's Assistant Deputy Ministers' Forum on Human Services. The objectives of the telecast were to: (1) address rewards and challenges of evaluating intersectoral programs, (2) facilitate sharing of ideas and experiences, (3) focus on common problems and solutions, (4) relate Saskatchewan experiences with evaluating intersectoral programs, and (5) introduce evaluation designs at multiple levels in a complex program.

The telecast was transmitted from the Saskatchewan Communications Network studio at the University of Saskatchewan to satellite reception sites in each of the thirty-two health districts in the province. Over six hundred people took part at these various locations.

Three major teaching and learning strategies were used to pursue the objectives of the conference. First, several groups across Saskatchewan took part in a pre-conference consultation process to identify critical issues in intersectoral evaluation. Second, presentations were broadcast from Saskatoon, and participants at all sites were able to submit questions by telephone and fax. The keynote speaker for the event was Michael Quinn Patton (independent evaluation consultant), and a number of panel presenters shared Saskatchewan experiences in evaluating intersectoral programs. Third, group discussions were facilitated at each of the sites.

The second of our large provincial events concerned the application of population health promotion approaches to the prevention of diabetes. The conference, entitled "Build Better Tomorrows: Work Together on the Determinants of Health," brought 314 participants together in Saskatoon from 12 to 14 February 2002. This conference was co-sponsored by Health Canada and Saskatchewan Health, and was planned by BHPC and representatives of the Battlefords Tribal Council, Canadian Diabetes Association, District Health Promotion Steering Group, Federation of Saskatchewan Indian Nations, Government of Saskatchewan's Human Services Integration Forum, Métis Nation of Saskatchewan, Prairie Region Health Promotion Research Centre, Prince Albert Grand Council, Saskatchewan Association of Health Organizations, and Saskatoon District Health. Given the focus of the conference, we recruited significant numbers of Aboriginal participants. The conference was designed to help participants: (1) learn about conditions that support health, (2) know what communities are doing to prevent diabetes, (3) learn the eight key population health promotion ideas, and (4) strengthen connections among health professionals.

In order to pursue these objectives, we used the pedagogical approach of our summer schools. That is, we blended plenary presentations from knowledgeable and credible resource people with facilitated small-group discussion sessions in which participants exchanged ideas and experiences over the course of the conference. The presentations involved panel discussions that illustrated key concepts of population health promotion in a variety of community action stories, plus the use of community examples from Saskatchewan and beyond. The small-group discussions focused on relating eight key population health promotion ideas to the plenary presentations and the experiences of the participants in each small group. The fact that the members of each small group met three times over the conference increased the network development impact of this event. Finally, we ensured that the conference included cultural activities of interest to Aboriginal people and opportunities for all participants to engage in social interaction and physical activity.

Complete results of the evaluation of this conference are available (Saskatchewan Heart Health Program 2002c). Most participants were satisfied with the event and believed that they had learned from taking part. In the follow-up evaluation, sixteen of eighteen respondents could identify specific examples of how they had subsequently applied what they had learned at the conference.

In summary, we delivered a substantial number and variety of continuing education events between 1998 and 2002. These events addressed, with diverse audiences, formats, and substantive foci, learning needs pertinent to building health promotion capacity across Saskatchewan. Our evaluation of these events indicates that a large number of health promotion practitioners were satisfied with the education they had received, had learned something about health promotion, and were able to integrate something of what they had learned into their professional practices.

Peer Networking (HPLINK)

Although we prided ourselves on the quality and innovative nature of our summer schools and other continuing education events, they involved relatively known and comfortable modes of action. Our third major form of intervention challenged those who took part in our work to use new information technologies to build capacity for health promotion work. At the beginning of BHPC, Health Canada supported our feasibility study into the potential of electronic networking to benefit the work of health promotion practitioners across Manitoba and Saskatchewan (Holmlund 1998). In late 1998, this study led to the formation of a working group to pilot and explore the usefulness of e-mail communication among health promotion practitioners in Saskatchewan. This working group was composed of seven Health Promotion Contacts, a Saskatchewan Health representative, and a staff member with BHPC. In the first half of 1999, this group exchanged regular messages, and established the foundation of what would become an e-mail listserv known as HPLINK. The listserv was formally launched at our summer school in August 1999. Its objectives were to: (1) mediate communication among practitioners of health promotion in Saskatchewan and beyond; (2) enable practitioners to communicate knowledge, insights, and creative solutions with others; and (3) share information and resources that practitioners found to be useful.

HPLINK was managed and facilitated by BHPC staff members (Bonnie Sproat and then Lorraine Khatchatourians), and was hosted by the University of Saskatchewan. Participation in HPLINK can be measured in two simple ways: the number of active subscribers to the list and the number of messages posted to the list by those subscribers. The number of subscribers gradually increased throughout the course of the BHPC project. In September 1999, there were 20 subscribers. The number doubled by December 1999, and reached 110 in October 2000. In August 2001, there were 121 subscribers, and this number climbed to 148 by July 2002 and 167 by February 2003.

The level of activity of these subscribers can be estimated in very crude terms by the number of postings to the listserv over time. We established HPLINK in the fall of 1999, and the number of messages sent increased from 263 in 2000 to 296 in 2001 and 343 in 2002. Table 4.3 provides basic data about the frequency of postings.

From an analysis of the archive of HPLINK, it is possible to determine who sent the messages counted in Table 4.3, what those messages were about, and the extent to which other subscribers responded to the messages. The complete archive is available at <http://www.usask.ca/lists/hplink>. In order to summarize the nature of postings to HPLINK, we selected seven months from the three-year history of the listerv and analyzed the number of messages posted according to the source, purpose, and topic. The data from this content analysis are presented in Tables 4.4 to 4.6.

The list manager sent most (66 percent) of the messages to HPLINK during these months. Most messages (64 percent) identified resources of potential benefit to health promotion practitioners. Other major purposes of messages to HPLINK were to share information about conferences or other educational opportunities (17 percent) and to pose questions about health promotion practice (5 percent). The thematic foci of messages to HPLINK varied greatly, with no single area accounting for more than 10 percent of the posted messages.

Beyond content analysis through the archival system of the listserv, we evaluated HPLINK through key informant interviews and a survey of subscribers to the list. A total of thirteen key informant interviews were conducted between December 2000 and March 2001. The informants included nine Health Promotion Contacts who were or had been subscribers to the list, three non-HPC subscribers, and the HPLINK list manager. In June 2001, we conducted an online survey of HPLINK subscribers to determine how people were using the listerv, how satisfied they were with it, and what their participation in HPLINK meant to their practice of health promotion. Forty subscribers responded to this survey, which amounts to a 35 percent response rate from the membership of 114 subscribers at the time.

Detailed results of our evaluation of HPLINK are available (Saskatchewan Heart Health Program 2002b). In summary, we can conclude that HPLINK has been a growing listserv for over three years. It has effectively disseminated information about health promotion to a significant number of health promotion practitioners, leaders, and scholars. HPLINK participants are reasonably satisfied with the listserv, and many

Table 4.3

Quarterly/average monthly postings to HPLINK, 2000-3

	1999	2000				2001				2002				2003
	Oct.-Dec.	Jan.-Mar.	Apr.-Jun.	Jul.-Sep.	Oct.-Dec.	Jan.-Mar.	Apr.-Jun.	Jul.-Sep.	Oct.-Dec.	Jan.-Mar.	Apr.-Jun.	Jul.-Sep.	Oct.-Dec.	Jan.-Mar.
	70/	72/	48/	55/	88/	86/	82/	70/	58/	85/	67/	62/	129/	127/
	23	24	16	18	29	29	27	23	19	28	22	21	43	42

Table 4.4

Number of messages posted to HPLINK, by source

Source	Month and year							
	Feb. 2000	Nov. 2000	Apr. 2001	Oct. 2001	May 2002	Sep. 2002	Jan. 2003	Total
List manager	6	17	26	14	16	23	35	137
Health district	2	0	1	0	5	2	2	12
Others	9	13	10	3	12	4	7	58
Total	17	30	37	17	33	29	44	207

Table 4.5

Number of messages posted to HPLINK, by purpose

Purpose of message	Month and year							Total
	Feb. 2000	Nov. 2000	Apr. 2001	Oct. 2001	May 2002	Sep. 2002	Jan. 2003	
Identifying Web-based resources	9	21	28	10	18	21	25	132
Conference announcements	0	3	6	4	4	4	15	36
Questions about practice	5	0	0	1	4	1	0	11
Other	3	6	3	2	7	3	4	28
Total	17	30	37	17	33	29	44	207

Table 4.6

Number of messages posted to HPLINK, by topic

Topic	Month and year							Total
	Feb. 2000	Nov. 2000	Apr. 2001	Oct. 2001	May 2002	Sep. 2002	Jan. 2003	
Child health	0	9	3	0	0	1	1	14
Community development	0	3	2	1	1	1	0	8
Diabetes	0	0	1	0	1	1	0	3
Education	5	0	2	2	2	1	8	20
Employment	0	0	0	1	1	1	0	3
Environment	0	0	2	0	0	1	1	4
Facilitation	3	0	0	0	0	0	1	4
General health promotion	1	3	0	1	6	0	2	13

▲

Topic	Month and year							
	Feb. 2000	Nov. 2000	Apr. 2001	Oct. 2001	May 2002	Sep. 2002	Jan. 2003	Total
Globalization	0	0	0	0	1	0	0	1
Health reform	0	0	1	1	0	0	1	3
Health economics	1	3	0	0	2	1	0	7
Health policy	0	1	5	1	1	4	3	15
Health ethics	0	0	0	0	0	0	2	2
HIV/AIDS	0	1	0	0	0	0	1	2
HPLINK	0	0	0	0	1	0	0	1
Humour	0	0	0	0	0	0	1	1
Injury	0	0	2	1	2	0	0	5
International development	1	0	0	0	0	0	1	2
Mental health	0	1	0	3	0	1	0	5
Nutrition	0	0	0	0	0	0	1	1
Organizational development	0	2	1	0	1	1	0	5
Physical activity	0	0	0	1	0	2	1	4
Population health	4	2	2	0	1	3	5	17
Poverty	0	1	1	1	5	1	2	11
Primary health	0	1	4	0	1	1	3	10
Program evaluation	0	0	1	2	2	3	1	9
Public health	0	2	1	0	0	0	2	5
Reproductive health	2	0	5	0	0	2	3	12
Rural health	0	0	0	1	0	0	0	1
Tobacco-related	0	0	1	0	3	1	4	9
Women's health	0	1	3	1	2	3	0	10
Total	17	30	37	17	33	29	44	207

have found it to be a source of learning and information resources to be shared with others. HPLINK has not flourished as an interactive networking medium, but it has been a useful source of information and a convenient portal to further resources. Subscribers have indicated that they appreciate the quality of information posted to HPLINK, and the fact that much information is screened and introduced with a short summary by the list manager.

Working with the Health Promotion Contacts

As discussed in Chapter 3, the Health Promotion Contacts played key roles in coordinating health promotion activities within their districts, and represented their districts to Saskatchewan Health on health promotion matters. In the design of the BHPC project, we conceptualized the HPCs as key agents of change in the health district system, and targeted many of our interventions toward them. We assumed that these individuals would be able to positively influence the evolution of their health districts' work in health promotion.

The HPCs were a diverse group of professionals. The 27 HPC respondents to our 1998 survey held a variety of different positions with the health districts. Twelve were employed as directors or coordinators of health promotion, 5 as community health educators, 5 as public health managers or nurses, 3 as directors of community services, and 1 each as social epidemiologist and public health nutritionist. Twenty-four of the HPCs were female. In terms of formal educational attainment, 5 had undergraduate certificates or diplomas, 17 had a bachelor's degree, and 5 had a master's degree. Fourteen HPCs were educated as nurses, 4 graduated from commerce programs, 4 from home economics programs, and 2 each from education and health sciences fields other than nursing. A total of 7 HPCs had additional, formal qualifications in health care administration.

In 1998, the HPCs had significant professional experience in the health and human services fields but they were fairly new to their roles within the health districts. Forty percent of the HPCs had served in their current position for less than eighteen months, and only 30 percent had done so for more than three years. In contrast, one-third of the HPCs had been employed in the health or human services sector for more than twenty years, and only one-fifth had less than three years of such experience. Sixty percent of the HPCs were in their thirties or forties, 20 percent were in their twenties, and 20 percent were in their fifties.

By 2000, there were modest changes in the demographic profile of the HPCs. Once again, only three HPCs were male. As could be expected, the HPCs were older and slightly more experienced, with two-thirds in their forties or fifties. The average length of time in their current position rose slightly (to just over 4 years), while the average length of service in the health or human services professions rose to just under 16.5 years. Staff turnover was significant in the HPC positions. Of the 22 health districts that completed the HPC Profile in 1998, 2000, and 2001, 7 (32 percent) had the same HPC respond to all three surveys, 11 (50 percent) had two HPCs respond to the three surveys, and 4 (18 percent) had three different HPCs respond. Of the 7 health districts that completed two HPC Profiles, 5 (71 percent) had two HPCs respond.

The HPCs were central to the BHPC project. On the one hand, they were integral to the success of our research practices. They were consulted in the development of our research instruments and data-gathering procedures. They were the respondents to our Health Promotion Contact Profile, and typically had a role in completing the Health District Capacity Survey. They were key informants in our effort to ensure that the work of BHPC was pertinent to the evolving circumstances of health districts across Saskatchewan. On the other hand, given the manner in which we had conceptualized them as change agents, the HPCs were a primary target audience for our educational interventions.

The HPCs from all Saskatchewan health districts met as a group on a more or less semi-annual schedule. Representatives of BHPC participated at HPC meetings on the following dates (the list also indicates the topics on which BHPC staff addressed the HPCs at those meetings):

- 15 June 1998, Introduction to Building Health Promotion Capacity
- 28 October 1998, Assessing Continuing Education Priorities
- 16 March 1999, Strategic Planning in the Health Districts
- 15 June 1999 (no BHPC session on the agenda)
- 18 October 1999, Update and Findings from BHPC
- 29 February 2000, Challenges in Facilitating Intersectoral Work
- 6 June 2000 (no BHPC session on the agenda)
- 3 October 2000, Update and Findings from BHPC
- 7 February 2001 (no BHPC session on the agenda)
- 17 October 2001, Organizational Capacity for Health Promotion
- 14 February 2002, Action Plan for Saskatchewan Health Care
- 22 May 2002, Organizational Capacity for Health Promotion: Learning from Practitioners

- 11 February 2003, Adult Education in Health Promotion Practice
- 12 February 2003, Update on the Evolution of BHPC

Health Promotion Contact meetings performed several functions. They were an opportunity for Saskatchewan Health staff to present new information or provide updates about provincial or national initiatives. They enabled various HPCs to showcase their health promotion projects. They encouraged networking, the sharing of resources and strategies, and the collaborative exploration of issues and priorities that affected many HPCs. Finally, they gave the HPCs the opportunity to discuss how to achieve systematic change to enhance the health promotion environment, or at least how to better cope within the existing environment.

BHPC staff played five roles at Health Promotion Contact meetings. They: (1) presented information about discrete issues in health promotion practice; (2) provided feedback with regard to the results of BHPC research processes; (3) listened to the HPCs and observed their interactions in order to remain grounded in the changing environment of health promotion practice; (4) asked reflective questions, posed issues for discussion, and provided BHPC's own observations about those questions and issues; and (5) offered technical advice during sessions, as well as at breaks and after the meetings.

These five roles were frequently interconnected. For example, when we presented our research results to the HPCs, we consistently structured a discussion with reflective questions. Such discussions frequently led to the identification of further learning needs, and this identification of needs influenced our subsequent provision of continuing education events at provincial and regional levels.

Ongoing involvement with the HPC meetings provided an informal means of validating our research findings and helped shape subsequent educational interventions. We did not formally evaluate our participation at the HPC meetings as a continuing education intervention, but we do have three indicators of the success of that participation. First, we were invited back to every HPC meeting over the course of the BHPC project, and were warmly received at those meetings. Second, we received numerous informal expressions of gratitude for the information and services provided at the HPC meetings. Third, we influenced the evolution of the format of the HPC meetings themselves. While initial meetings were often a series of lectures with modest time for questions, later meetings involved the more creative use of effective adult education principles in providing information.

Educating Health District Leaders

We conceptualized the Health Promotion Contacts as key agents of change within the health district system. However, we also believed that capacity for health promotion action could be built only within a supportive environment. Leadership provided by senior and middle managers (such as health district chief executive officers and community service managers) and elected or appointed officials (such as health district board members) helped shape health promotion practice. We therefore made regular efforts to educate health district leaders about health promotion, and to advocate for a commitment to supporting health promotion throughout their organizations.

The first manner in which we tried to influence health district leaders was through making presentations at conferences and orientation sessions at which such leaders gathered. Each year, the Saskatchewan Association of Health Organizations (SAHO) organizes a conference attended by many health district CEOs, senior managers, and board members. For three years, BHPC representatives gave workshops at these conferences:

- 22 March 1999, Partnering for Action on Health Determinants: Making It Happen (270 participants in two sessions)
- 20 March 2000, We're Drowning: Turn Off the Tap! (190 participants)
- 19 March 2001, Does Health Promotion Work? How Do We Know? (55 participants)

Further, at the SAHO board orientation session on 29 November 2001, we gave a presentation entitled "Building Health" to about seventy-five participants.

Our 1999 SAHO presentation endeavoured to build health district leaders' awareness of how to engage in partnerships to take action on the determinants of health. The objectives of our session were to: (1) explore case examples of health districts taking action on health determinants, and (2) identify lessons about dealing with the challenges of addressing basic health determinants through intersectoral action.

We argued that if health districts were to go beyond the treatment of illness to address the social, economic, and environmental issues that determine a population's health, they needed to develop partnerships with other organizations and agencies that were also dealing with health determinants. Such partnerships were presented as an effective means of countering the common lament that health districts did not have the resources or authority to address or control the issues outside the health care system that affect health. Four presenters with pertinent experience provided examples of how strategic partnerships can promote effective action on a range of health determinants. A panel of three discussants then identified insights into ways of building and sustaining these important partnerships and strategies.

Our 2000 SAHO presentation was intended to educate health district leaders about health promotion capacity and capacity building. Our objectives were to: (1) raise awareness about health promotion and the components of health promotion capacity; (2) encourage sharing of ideas and strategies about capacity building; and (3) introduce the BHPC "Organizational Health Promotion Capacity Checklist" (see Chapter 8) as a potential tool for fostering awareness, discussion, and change. We used plenary presentations and small-group discussions to engage district leaders in an exploration of health promotion capacity: what it means, why it is important, and how to strengthen it.

Our 2001 SAHO presentation focused on identifying ways to make evidence-based, informed decisions for effective health promotion investments. We focused on the evidence for the effectiveness of health promotion, and on ways in which health district boards could support health promotion activities. Our presentation at this board orientation sought to sensitize new health district board members to the importance and key issues in population health promotion. Its objectives were to help participants understand: (1) the evidence for the effectiveness of health promotion, (2) the essential elements of a population health promotion approach, (3) the factors promoting and hindering health promotion capacity at the health district level, and (4) the ways in which health district boards can respond to the challenges of becoming more involved in health promotion. Our presentation involved a conceptual introduction to population health promotion as well as a case study of actions taken by one health district to support health promotion.

The second manner in which we tried to influence health district leaders consisted of providing information about the BHPC project and engaging such leaders in our research processes. In April 1998, we sent a letter to each health district CEO. This letter described the BHPC project and highlighted the importance of health promotion capacity for health districts. In August 1998, we sent a second letter, asking for health districts to volunteer to become "case study" or "case monitoring" districts (see Chapter 3). Fourteen of thirty health districts volunteered to serve in this capacity. District CEOs received each of our three Health District Capacity Surveys. In January 2000, we made three presentations to provincial gatherings of key health district leaders: the chief executive officers, the medical health officers, and the community service directors.

We made subsequent presentations to the medical health officers on 14 February 2000 and to the community service directors on 23 January 2002. These presentations reviewed research findings from the BHPC project, and also served as an opportunity for education and advocacy with regard to health promotion.

The third manner in which we tried to influence health district leaders consisted of facilitating an organizational development learning circle. The learning circle was accomplished through a series of events developed with and for a group of health promotion practitioners and leaders with selected health districts across the province. Our aim was to find a way to support personnel in health districts in understanding, articulating, and planning for meeting the challenges of integrating health promotion more fully into their organizations. This included developing a better organizational climate for health promotion, and broadening or deepening the organization's understanding of principles and strategies of population health promotion. We proposed that this also included being or becoming a learning organization and a healthy organization. To accomplish this objective, we invited practitioners to join us in a learning circle. A learning circle is a group that shares the tasks of bringing information to the group, working together to understand the information, bringing experience into the circle, and coming away more aware and confident.

The organizational development learning circle met four times over the course of four months in late 2001 and early 2002. The participants were thirteen leaders from health districts across the province. They were deliberately chosen to represent a diversity of managerial positions responsible for a variety of services. Six staff members of BHPC also took part.

The first meeting of the learning circle took place on 3 October 2001 in Saskatoon. The objectives of this half-day workshop were to: (1) begin the process of learning together (i.e., to form a learning circle), (2) develop a sense of shared reality and of how we could support each other, (3) identify factors and strategies that either facilitate or impede organizational capacity development, and (4) explore the use of guided imagery and the story-dialogue method for analyzing and understanding personal experiences with organizational change.

The two major processes used to structure this workshop were guided imagery and the story-dialogue method. The guided imagery exercise enabled participants to reflect upon a concrete personal experience in which they had been agents of change in an organization. The story-dialogue method enabled them to gather and analyze detailed case studies of developing organizational capacity for health promotion.

The second event in the organizational development learning circle took place on 21 October 2001 in Saskatoon. Unlike the other three events, it was not a meeting dedicated to the learning circle itself. Rather, it was a pre-conference workshop, sponsored by BHPC, in conjunction with the annual conference of the Canadian Public Health Association. The one-day workshop, "Creating Conditions for Health-Promoting Organizations: A Five-Step Model," was facilitated by Dr. Harvey Skinner (University of Toronto, Department of Public Health Sciences) and Pearl Bader (Ontario Centre for Addiction and Mental Health). The objectives of the workshop were to: (1) understand how organizational factors influence both practitioners and clients/patients in prevention, health promotion, and behavioural health care; (2) provide skill-based learning in applying the Five-Step Model and Tools for organizational improvement; and (3) stimulate ongoing professional development regarding organizational change. The workshop involved presentations from the facilitators as well as small-group discussion and role-playing activities.

The third event in the organizational development learning circle took place on 30 November 2001 in Saskatoon. Besides learning circle participants, the following guests participated:

- April Barry, Population Health Promotion Branch, Saskatchewan Health
- John Carter, Saskatchewan Association of Health Organizations
- Dennis Chubb, Regional Intersectoral Committee on Human Services Coordinator
- Kathy GermAnn, graduate student, University of Alberta
- Dennis Moore, District Management Services Branch, Saskatchewan Health

The objectives of this full-day workshop were to: (1) continue the process of learning together and supporting each other, (2) articulate what we had learned so far and what we wanted to learn, and (3) identify next steps in developing our capacity to be change agents.

In this workshop, the process of being an effective agent of change for organizational development in health promotion was described as having three simple domains: understanding (knowing how organizations change), analyzing (examining particular organizations to determine how to make change), and doing (planning, undertaking, and evaluating processes of change). Participants in the learning circle identified what they had already learned and what they still needed to know about these domains of being change agents in organizations. This workshop generated many ideas about how to build effective health promotion organizations.

The fourth event in the organizational development learning circle took place on 22 January 2003 in Regina. It was not initially part of the learning-circle process but was added in response to requests from participants at the 30 November event. The objectives of this meeting were to: (1) examine the concept of change and tools for analyzing change; (2) debrief changes resulting from announcement of the Action Plan for Saskatchewan Health Care; (3) share experiences and insights, to keep participants grounded in the face of change; and (4) make decisions regarding the future of the group, and future steps needed to build organizational capacity for health promotion.

This meeting included a presentation about the theories of organizational change and a facilitated discussion of the next steps in becoming more effective agents of change, both individually and collectively, in the contemporary health promotion environment in Saskatchewan.

It was difficult to measure the success of our efforts to educate health district leaders about health promotion. The extent of our engagement with those leaders was typically much lower than the extent of our engagement with health promotion practitioners. We were able to spend less time with them, and we were not able to evaluate the outcomes of that time as closely as we could with the practitioners. The organizational development learning circle was well received by its participants, but because it took place at the same time as a major restructuring of the health district system, it is very difficult to know what contribution the learning circle may have made to leaders' efforts to guide or adapt to that restructuring.

Consultation, Networking, and Advocacy
In addition to the five major interventions that have been described in this chapter, we made a variety of more modest contributions to building capacity for health promotion in Saskatchewan. These contributions took place through consulting services, support to existing networks, and advocacy with Saskatchewan Health.

Consulting Services
BHPC staff members were available as consultants to practitioners and

health districts for various forms of support and capacity development. While our modest human resources dedicated to consulting services precluded us from assertively marketing such services, we did make use of a toll-free number to encourage calls from across the province. Requests for consulting services were not consistently monitored over the course of the project. Team members were more likely to create records of calls that were of interest because of the challenge inherent in the subject matter, because there could be significant implications for the team in other aspects of the project, or because the call in some way reflected on previous actions of the team.

Based on seventy-two recorded requests for consultation, we can offer the following description of the consulting services we provided over the course of the project. Just over half of the requests came from health district staff. Requests came for three basic types of services: for advice or support, for someone to work with an individual or group, and for workshops or training sessions. More specifically, we received and recorded the following broad categories of requests, in descending order of frequency:

- Advice/technical help with *practice issues* or situations (19)
- Advice/technical help with *applied research* problems (11)
- Advice/technical help with *training or professional development* challenges (11)
- Request for someone to *facilitate a group process* (7)
- Request for a *workshop/training session* (6)
- Request for someone to *do applied research* (5)
- Request for someone to *do program evaluation* (4)
- Request for someone to *speak at a meeting* or conference (4)
- Request for *evidence* on the effectiveness of health promotion (3)
- Request for *support, affirmation, validation, and encouragement* (2)

We responded in various ways, according to the nature of the request. When advice or support was requested, team members listened, engaged in dialogue, shared insights, and offered encouragement. As appropriate, consultants would send written resources and/or suggest others who could be contacted for specific forms of assistance. Requests for someone to help a group with a process or problem were more challenging to the team. Given the other commitments and demands of the project, it was usually not possible for team members to take on extensive consulting work. However, consultants would discuss each problem, suggest approaches, and refer the request to one or more individuals known to the team to do good work in the relevant areas.

Early in the program, we determined that wherever patterns were observable among the requests for consultation, consideration would be given to developing a broader response to the field as a whole, for the sake of economy of effort and to achieve maximum impact. We interpreted requests for "someone to do for us" as often an indication of lack of capacity within the organization making the request. We were highly conscious of the need to avoid "doing for" and thereby creating dependence or undermining capacity. Instead, we would examine how to respond to the need through training on a more universal basis. So, for example, inquiries about program evaluation support persistently indicated need for program evaluation training, which was incorporated into the curricula of summer schools.

The nature of requests for consulting services changed over time. Most categories or types of request were represented in all years of the consultation service, but requests for workshops tended to cluster in the first three years. During those years, BHPC was active in providing workshops, which in turn gave rise to requests for either further training for groups requesting it or similar training for another target audience. As summer schools became better targeted to the needs of practitioners, requests for training workshops could be referred to the upcoming summer schools. Requests in the early years of the program were somewhat more likely to be for basic information or to reflect a need for introduction to the field of health promotion. In later years, the requests reflected increased sophistication (e.g., for facilitation of a session on health promotion capacity development; for advice on how to evaluate a multilevel program; for advice on how to advertise for a health promotion specialist with high individual capacity, and how to provide a rich organizational environment for that practitioner).

Support to Existing Networks
The BHPC project actively participated in the Saskatchewan Population Health Promotion Partnership (SPHPP) throughout the period 1998-2003. This partnership had been created in 1996 with PRHPRC as prime mover, along with Saskatchewan Health's Population Health Branch and Health Canada's Health Promotion and Programs Branch (Manitoba/Saskatchewan Region). By 1998, the group had grown to include the Saskatchewan Association of Health Organizations, Human Services Integration Forum, Métis Family and Community Justice, Federation of Saskatchewan Indian Nations, Saskatchewan Indian Federated College, Saskatchewan Health District Management Services Branch, Saskatch-

ewan Public Health Association, and the District Health Promotion Steering Group. SPHPP defined itself as a coalition formed to support and strengthen population health promotion in Saskatchewan. It facilitated coordinated planning by developing mutual support, fostering skill development, and disseminating and communicating information.

In 1998, Joan Feather invited SPHPP to act as an informal provincial advisory committee to assist BHPC in monitoring needs and developments in the health promotion field in the province, including but not limited to the developments in the health districts. SPHPP readily agreed. Throughout the BHPC project, Joan continued to report on the progress of BHPC and to bring the BHPC perspective to SPHPP in its environmental scanning and strategic planning. SPHPP typically met two or three times per year, often for two-day retreats.

Involvement in SPHPP gave BHPC a larger role in creating synergy among organizations and groups sharing the goal of building health promotion capacity in the province. There were reciprocal benefits for BHPC and SPHPP. Because of the research dimension of the BHPC project, BHPC involvement in SPHPP significantly strengthened the information base on which SPHPP established its strategic plans. In turn, SPHPP facilitated formation of groups of interested stakeholders for continuing education events (e.g., summer school planning), helped publicize training events and resources arising from BHPC, provided advice on opportunities and strategic choices for continuing education and networking activities of BHPC, and helped create a rich and supportive environment for practitioners.

Advocacy and Capacity Building within Saskatchewan Health
As explained in Chapter 2, close, cooperative relations between PRHPRC and Saskatchewan Health's Population Health Branch predated the BHPC project. In addition, the Branch had been a supportive partner in previous phases of the Saskatchewan Heart Health Program (SHHP). Saskatchewan Health agreed to play a key role in the BHPC project through the appointment of the provincial Chief Medical Health Officer (David Butler-Jones) as one of the co-principal investigators, and through the provision of $75,000 per year for five years.

We recognized the key role played by the Branch in providing support and resources directly to the practitioners whose capacity we aimed to enhance, and therefore took every available opportunity to include Branch staff in our capacity development initiatives, as colleagues, collaborators, and learners. For example, the Branch consistently provided funding and planning group members for summer schools. It also registered numerous staff in those summer schools. There were informal consultations between BHPC and Branch staff throughout the program to exchange ideas, assess opportunities, explore learning needs, and coordinate shared initiatives.

We have anecdotal evidence of the positive impact of BHPC on the skills and knowledge of Population Health Branch staff and their capacity to design and promote population health promotion initiatives. One example of this impact, as identified by Branch staff, concerned their design and implementation of a provincial initiative called the Population Health Promotion Demonstration Projects for the Prevention of Diabetes. This initiative was designed to encourage communities and health districts to engage in effective intersectoral actions on the primary prevention of Type II diabetes, and also to build understanding and capacity for population health promotion in general. The designers drew on tools and processes for planning, program design, evaluation, and formation of effective intersectoral partnerships that had been the focus of BHPC summer schools. They developed training workshops for district staff and other sector partners, incorporating aspects of the learning designs and practices of the summer schools and BHPC workshops. The health district staff who participated were quick to recognize the synergy that had been created between Saskatchewan Health and BHPC. Further, the provincial initiative offered funding to create opportunities for practitioners to apply the learning from summer schools and other BHPC training events.

Conclusion

In this chapter, we have described the major actions we took to facilitate the learning of others. We have described our summer schools and the other provincial or regional continuing education events through which we endeavoured to enhance the knowledge, skills, and commitment of a broad range of health promotion practitioners. We have narrated our efforts to establish a listserv to promote better communication among health promotion practitioners. We have discussed the efforts made to provide information and educational opportunities to Health Promotion Contacts and health district leaders. It is important to note that while these interventions have been presented in separate sections, they were in fact interrelated. For example, our meetings with the Health Promotion Contacts often led to ideas or invitations to deliver or adapt continuing education events.

Figure 4.1

Summary of capacity-building interventions

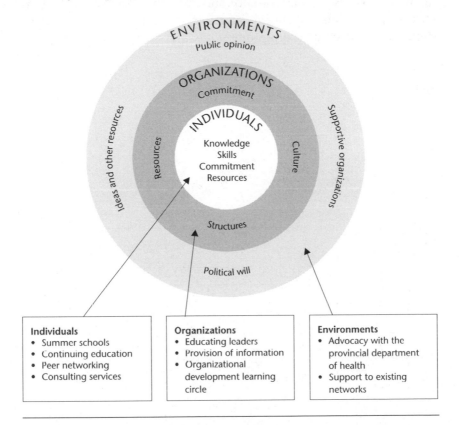

Individuals	**Organizations**	**Environments**
• Summer schools	• Educating leaders	• Advocacy with the
• Continuing education	• Provision of information	provincial department
• Peer networking	• Organizational	of health
• Consulting services	development learning	• Support to existing
	circle	networks

From taking action to facilitate the learning of health promotion practitioners and leaders, we learned a great deal about health promotion
capacity and its development. What we learned from this action is the
focus of the next three chapters. Figure 4.1 both foreshadows those chapters and summarizes the interventions we carried out to build health
promotion capacity among practitioners and organizations.

Figure 4.1 identifies the basic elements of health promotion capacity
among individuals and organizations, as well as the key characteristics
of environments supportive of such capacity. Through summer schools
and other continuing education events, peer networking, and consulting services, we endeavoured to build the knowledge, skills, and commitment of health promotion practitioners. Through education,

information provision, and a learning circle, we endeavoured to enhance the organizational commitment, structures, culture, and investment of resources in health promotion. Through advocacy and support of existing networks, we endeavoured to create a more supportive environment for effective health promotion work.

Part 3
Learning from Action

5
Practitioners

The Building Health Promotion Capacity (BHPC) project involved considerable action for learning. We organized, delivered, and evaluated a substantial number of continuing education opportunities for health promotion practitioners. We engaged such practitioners in a range of research processes designed to learn about the nature of health promotion capacity and the manner in which such capacity evolves. From this action, two main types of learning took place. First, we learned something about capacity, how it evolves over time, and how it can be nurtured through continuing education practice. Second, the health promotion practitioners with whom we worked learned about health promotion and how to engage in it effectively. In this chapter, we describe this learning according to three guiding questions:

- What elements constitute the capacity of individuals to engage in effective health promotion action?
- How does such capacity develop over time?
- What capacity development was experienced by the health promotion practitioners with whom we worked?

Before exploring these questions, we need to state one caveat: health promotion practitioners have a broad range of experiences, responsibilities, and approaches to practice. The following list exemplifies the range of health promotion roles taken on by various practitioners with whom we worked: (1) providing health education in clinical and community settings; (2) planning, delivering, and evaluating community-based programs; (3) advocating for health promotion at organizational and political levels; (4) educating colleagues about health promotion practices; (5) engaging individuals and groups in community development processes; and (6) building partnerships with other practitioners, organizations, and communities.

Given the diversity of what it means to actually practise health promotion, it would be futile to seek a universal account of what constitutes capacity, or how to develop capacity, among all health promotion practitioners. Our exploration of health promotion capacity is grounded in experience with practitioners and organizations in Saskatchewan from 1998 to 2003. We will present an account of health promotion capacity and capacity development that is definitive enough to be meaningful but open-ended enough to respect the diversity that characterizes the activities in which health promotion practitioners engage.

The Nature of Health Promotion Capacity at the Individual Level

Individual capacity to engage in effective health promotion activities is composed of elements of knowledge, skills, commitment, and resources. Figure 5.1 indicates the main elements of capacity that we have identified as important for health promotion practitioners.

Knowledge

There is a knowledge base upon which effective health promotion practice is constructed. This knowledge base begins with a holistic understanding of health and its determinants. Health, of course, is more than the absence of disease. The Saskatchewan Provincial Health Council (1994) defined health as "a dynamic process involving the harmony of physical, mental, emotional, social and spiritual well-being. Health enables individuals, families and communities to function to the best of their ability within their environment." The notion of "determinants of health" refers to the range of influences that combine to predispose individuals (and populations) to different states of health (see Chapter 2).

Population health promotion is a way of working to address the determinants of health among individuals, families, and communities. We have worked with Saskatchewan Health to define eight principles of the population health promotion approach: (1) meaningful participation of those whose health is being promoted; (2) action on a variety of health determinants; (3) collaboration and partnerships beyond the health care sector; (4) policy development to nurture environments that support healthy choices; (5) capacity building and empowerment; (6) actions that focus on the health of populations, not individuals; (7) working "upstream" (on the root causes of issues or problems); and (8) evidence-based decision making.

Figure 5.1

The basic elements of practitioners' health promotion capacity

Category	Basic elements of capacity
Knowledge	• A holistic understanding of health and its determinants • An awareness of population health promotion principles • An understanding of a variety of strategies and processes through which effective health promotion interventions can be undertaken • A recognition of the contextual specificity of the strengths and weaknesses of different health promotion strategies and processes • A familiarity with the conditions, aspirations, and culture of the population(s) with which one works
Skills	• Program planning (needs assessment, design, implementation, and evaluation) • Communication across sectors, disciplines, and socio-economic or community boundaries • Working with others (e.g., nurturing relationships, participation, and intersectoral partnerships; facilitation; conflict mediation) • Integrating research and practice (both in the program planning cycle and as a means of critically reflective practice) • Capacity building (both within one's own organization and with the external communities and organizations with which one works) • Being strategic and selective in making decisions about what to do and how to do it
Commitment	• Personal energy, enthusiasm, patience, and persistence • Values of population health promotion • Willingness to be flexible, to innovate, and to take thoughtful risks • Learning from experience of oneself and others • Self-confidence and credibility • Believing in and advocating for health promotion
Resources	• Time to engage in health promotion practice and in personal and professional development that enhances such practice • Tools for more efficient and effective practice, including resource inventories and repertoires of good ideas and best practices • Infrastructure, including office space, capital equipment, and effective means of communication • Supportive managers, colleagues, and allies with whom to work and learn • Access to adequate funding for health promotion activities

Given these principles, there is a range of strategies and processes through which effective health promotion interventions can be undertaken. Effective health promotion practice requires an understanding of different approaches and how to use them, as well as the recognition that the strengths and weaknesses of different approaches make them more or less appropriate in different circumstances. The following strategies can be used to influence the determinants of health: (1) health education at the individual level, (2) public awareness and social marketing, (3) small-group development, (4) mutual support or self-help activities, (5) coalition building (including intersectoral partnerships), (6) community organizing or community development, (7) public policy development or advocacy, and (8) social change movements and political activism.

To know which of these strategies to use in any given situation requires more than an abstract awareness of the strategies themselves; it requires familiarity with the conditions, aspirations, and culture of the people with whom one works. In other words, the knowledge base of effective health promotion practice moves beyond the principles and strategies of health promotion and includes practical knowledge of the context within which such principles and strategies will be employed. Understanding the context of one's work and being familiar with a range of health promotion strategies enable practitioners to select strategies that are suited to the contexts and challenges with which they are working.

Skills
Health promotion is a practical art, requiring more than simply knowledge. Practitioners must be able to actually get things done in the world. Figure 5.1 identifies six sets of skills required for effective health promotion practice. These skill sets are not specific to the practice of health promotion, but rather are important to a range of human and social service professions. Given that they are widely known, we do not elaborate on them here.

Commitment
Health promotion practice takes more than simply knowledge and skills. To be an effective practitioner also requires a set of personal qualities that we have termed "commitment," but that others might recognize as attitudes or dispositions. The first element of such commitment is a complex set of personal qualities that involves energy, enthusiasm, patience, and persistence. Personal energy and enthusiasm are obviously important to any profession that involves intense and challenging work

with people. The nature of health promotion work makes such qualities even more important. Effective health promotion practitioners tend to view their work as more than just a job. Health promotion is a vocation (something worthy of pursuit for its intrinsic value) as much as it is a profession. Energy and enthusiasm need to be matched with patience and persistence, given the long-range commitment needed for effective health promotion.

Second, health promotion capacity involves a belief in a series of values that define a way of acting in the world. Although such values may be hard to enumerate in a comprehensive and mutually exclusive manner, the following list represents values that are widely shared by the population health promotion community: (1) equity and social justice, (2) empowerment and participation, (3) cooperation and collective action, and (4) respect for human diversity and the natural environment.

Such values form an important set of assumptions about how health promotion practice should be carried out. Personal commitment to such values provides a framework for decision making amid the constantly shifting landscape of programs, projects, and funding opportunities that define much day-to-day health promotion work.

Third, health promotion capacity involves a willingness to be flexible, to innovate, and to take risks. No one approach to health promotion could possibly be suited to addressing all health determinants in all settings. Practitioners therefore need to be flexible and willing to adopt approaches suited to different challenges. Sometimes this will require innovation and a willingness to take risks. In taking risks, mistakes will be made, and effective practitioners must be prepared to accept such mistakes and learn from them. The commitment to learn from experience is a fourth personal characteristic of effective health promotion practitioners. The critically reflective practitioner is constantly learning, both from his or her own experiences and from the experiences that others share through publications, presentations, and less formal discussions. The commitment to learning is a key element of capacity for health promotion because it ensures that such capacity will be sustained and developed over time.

Fifth, health promotion capacity involves self-confidence and personal credibility. Self-confidence and credibility are really markers as much as they are elements of capacity. When a practitioner has the knowledge, skills, and commitment to undertake effective health promotion work, that individual is much more likely to have the confidence to undertake new and challenging forms of such work. Confidence in one's own capacity for health promotion is related in part to the confidence that others have of one's capacity. In other words, the internal sense of oneself as a competent practitioner is supported by the external affirmation of one's competence by others. Thus, the personal credibility of health promotion practitioners is both rooted in one's past actions and causally linked to the effectiveness of one's actions in the future. The processes of building capacity, self-confidence, and personal credibility are interconnected: improvement in one of these areas fosters and supports the enhancement of the others. Confidence and credibility are linked to one's ability and willingness to serve as an advocate for health promotion.

Resources
Individual capacity for health promotion involves the knowledge, skills, and commitment required to engage in health promotion activities. Through knowledge, practitioners know what to do. Through skills, they are able to take action. Through commitment, they find ways to act, even in the face of adverse circumstances. The operationalization of knowledge, skills, and commitment is facilitated by the access of individuals to resources for health promotion practice. While not a characteristic of individuals, resources are so closely tied to the ability of practitioners to translate their capacities into actions that we have identified five resources as elements of individual capacity for health promotion action. As with our discussion of skills, there is little need to elaborate on the resources listed in Figure 5.1. Time, tools, infrastructure, allies, and funding are needed in many fields other than health promotion, and the ability of practitioners to access such resources has a clear impact on their capacity to plan, implement, and evaluate health promotion activities.

Limits to the Efficacy of Individual Capacity
The capacity of individual practitioners to undertake health promotion activities is influenced by factors over which they have limited control. These factors are determined both by the characteristics of the organizations with which the practitioners work and by the social environment in which the practitioners and their organizations exist. Of course, the availability of resources identified in Figure 5.1 constitutes the most immediate constraint to the realization of practitioners' capacity. However, beyond such immediate resources, organizational and environmental factors mediate the extent to which individual capacity is translated into effective health promotion action. Since Chapter 6 will address organizational capacity and Chapter 7 will address environmen-

tal influences on health promotion capacity, we will not review these factors here. At this point, it is simply important to recognize that individual capacity for health promotion does not translate directly into effective health promotion action.

The Development of Health Promotion Capacity

Key Factors and Processes

In practical terms, a key reason to understand health promotion capacity is to be able to systematically help practitioners become more effective. The capacity of individuals to practice health promotion is constituted by the complex range of elements identified in Figure 5.1. Logically, the development of individual capacity would seem to be a simple process of enhancing the knowledge, skills, commitment, and resources of the practitioner such that he or she is better prepared to engage in health promotion action. In the real world, however, the linear progression toward greater capacity is very often made complex by the nature of individuals and their organizations. While capacity development should ideally involve the progressive building of greater capacity within each of the elements of capacity we have defined, this was not the experience of the practitioners with whom we worked. The history of capacity development among these practitioners was more complex than some logical progression toward a predetermined goal of greater capacity.

Capacity development among health promotion practitioners is an idiosyncratic process. Every individual has a life history. The capacity of each individual reflects a broad range of experiences, many of which have nothing to do with the intentional pursuit of health promotion capacity. Unintentional experiences that strongly influence one's capacity for health promotion work include such things as early childhood experiences, formative personal relationships, schooling, and initial training in professions or trades that may or may not bear close resemblance to health promotion. As a result, there are nearly as many capacity-building stories as there are practitioners. Even in terms of the limited realm of intentional efforts to build capacity, there is no single path toward becoming an effective health promotion practitioner. We cannot even make the same kind of generalizations about health promotion practitioners that we might be able to make about physicians, where the initial education and certification process leads to a certain standardization of educational and experiential backgrounds.

On the one hand, fully understanding the development of health promotion capacity in any given practitioner requires attention to the complex life history of that practitioner. On the other hand, such attention is of limited practical value. Formative experiences and unintentional biographical details are important to a rich understanding of an individual's capacity; however, they can be treated as more or less randomly distributed background variables when trying to understand and promote the capacity of a sufficiently large group of practitioners. If the practical goal is to systematically enhance the capacity of health promotion practitioners, then it is important to understand common patterns in the seemingly idiosyncratic experiences of individuals.

We argue that, despite the complexity and diversity of health promotion capacity among individual practitioners, a relatively small number of factors tend to catalyze capacity-building processes. In the experience of the practitioners with whom we worked, individual capacity was nurtured by: (1) the support of management and colleagues within the health district; (2) undertaking new roles and responsibilities; (3) the opportunity to encounter new ideas and practices through means such as continuing education, networking, and resource materials; and (4) the timely opportunity to apply newly encountered knowledge, and practise newly acquired skills in significant projects and partnerships.

Management support was critical to the availability of time and other resources for practitioners to actually engage in health promotion. As an element of organizational capacity, management support will be discussed in the next chapter. The support of colleagues was a two-sided coin for health promotion practitioners. On one side of the coin, ideas and resources obtained through working with supportive colleagues were often a catalyst to greater capacity. On the other side, non-supportive colleagues could result in isolation, obstructionism, and even the sabotage of health promotion initiatives. Absence of support was sometimes experienced as a simple lack of awareness or understanding of health promotion, and sometimes as a more complex form of hostility rooted in territoriality or "turf protection." In organizational settings in which health promotion was emerging at the same time as overall resources were perceived to be shrinking, new health promotion initiatives did not always get a friendly reception. Support of management and colleagues was fundamental to the development of greater health promotion capacity among practitioners. Such support was an important precursor to each of the other three catalysts to capacity development.

Individual capacity was nurtured by undertaking new roles and responsibilities. For some practitioners, taking on a new position created a need to learn more about health promotion or to engage in health promotion work at a new level. The experience of such engagement translated into new knowledge, skills, and a stronger commitment to health promotion. Interestingly, some practitioners who came to health promotion roles from acute care or clinical service backgrounds actually saw their previous experience as a great advantage in health promotion work. The advantage was rooted both in enhanced credibility in the eyes of health district colleagues and the general public, and in a stronger ability to make connections between health promotion activities and clinical health outcomes. Changing jobs was not always involved in the assumption of new responsibilities. Some practitioners took on significant new responsibilities within the context of an existing position. Practitioners identified the assumption of responsibility for initiatives such as major public relations campaigns and accreditation processes as important catalysts to the development of their capacity for health promotion work. Whether through a new position or an expanded set of responsibilities, learning on the job was often central to the enhancement of individuals' health promotion capacity.

Individual capacity was nurtured by the opportunity to encounter new ideas and practices through means such as continuing education, networking, and the availability of resource materials. Chapter 4 illustrated how continuing education and networking led to learning and behavioural change among health promotion practitioners. In general terms, continuing education and networking led to the development of health promotion capacity through four major pathways:

- *immediately applicable knowledge or skills,* when lessons learned through continuing education or networking were quickly translated into new health promotion practices
- *latent knowledge or skills,* when lessons learned through continuing education or networking were not quickly put into practice, but nevertheless enhanced the confidence and capacity of practitioners to act at a later date
- *perspective making,* when lessons learned through continuing education or networking were linked to an overall change of commitment or understanding that was relevant to a wide variety of future practices
- *team building,* when continuing education and networking events had the effect of bringing together and strengthening working groups that would later practise health promotion together

Through these pathways, continuing education and networking acted as catalysts to the development of capacity among individual health promotion practitioners.

Individual capacity was nurtured by the timely opportunity to apply newly encountered knowledge and practise newly acquired skills in significant projects and partnerships. The role of meaningful projects and partnerships in the development of capacity will be discussed more fully in the next chapter (since this role is essentially parallel for organizations and individuals), but it is important to state here that isolated continuing education events had a limited impact on capacity development. The evaluation of our continuing education initiatives consistently indicated that learning at educational events was most effectively translated into behavioural change in practice settings when there were opportunities to apply what was learned. Indeed, the gap between the excitement of new learning and the reality of long-term capacity change was often explained by the absence of meaningful opportunities to put new learning into practice. New knowledge and skills were not the only catalysts to capacity development; practice opportunities could also be useful in reinforcing existing knowledge or nurturing latent skills that had never been sufficiently mastered.

Intentionally Shaping Experiences for Capacity Building
Although capacity may be developed without explicit effort to do so, it is possible to nurture capacity among practitioners by engaging them in learning processes. Individual capacity to engage in effective health promotion activities may be nurtured through a cyclical process of continuing education, practical experience, and critical reflection. The first phase of this cycle is essentially bringing people into contact with new knowledge and skills. Through on-the-job experiences, continuing education, networking, or independent access to information, capacity development begins when individuals encounter ideas that make them consider how they currently understand and practise health promotion. The second phase of this cycle is essentially structuring the opportunity for application of new knowledge and skills. Through on-the-job experiences or simulations achieved through strategies such as role playing or internships, capacity development takes root when individuals experiment with actually practising health promotion in a different way. The third phase of this cycle is essentially the integration of action and awareness. Through disciplined and critical reflection, capacity development is integrated into long-term personal commitment when individuals relate new experiences and ideas to previously existing patterns of thought and practice.

The identification of the cyclical nature of capacity building makes clear demands on the organization for effective continuing education or staff development programs. Such programs must be more than simply the transmission of new ideas or the assignment of new duties. Rather, new ideas must be systematically linked to the opportunity to apply those ideas in a meaningful setting. New ideas and experiences must be integrated into existing structures of meaning and action through active and critical reflection.

We have illustrated that the development of health promotion capacity among individual practitioners is a complex and diverse process. There is no single pathway to capacity: many of the experiences that lead to capacity are unintentional, and many of the factors that help or hinder capacity building are beyond the control of the practitioners themselves. This does not mean that intentional and directed efforts to develop capacity are therefore futile. On the contrary, our findings confirm that individual capacity to engage in effective health promotion activities may be nurtured through a cyclical process of continuing education, practical experience, and critical reflection.

Capacity Building through the BHPC Project
Intentionally shaping experiences for capacity building was perhaps the single biggest task of the BHPC program. In Chapter 4, we described the interventions that we organized from 1998 through 2003 in order to build health promotion capacity in Saskatchewan. We demonstrated that many participants in BHPC continuing education events developed their health promotion capacity, and subsequently changed their health promotion practice, as a result of what they learned at those events. Based on our experience, we believe that carefully designed and delivered continuing education can make a significant contribution to capacity development. This belief is grounded in an extended dialogue that we undertook, through surveys and interviews, with Health Promotion Contacts (HPCs) across Saskatchewan.

Most HPCs experienced some capacity development over the course of the BHPC project. From their responses to closed-ended survey questions, we know that on average the HPCs believed that their knowledge, skills, and overall health promotion capacity improved a modest amount in the years 1999 and 2000. We asked the HPCs to respond to the questions, "To what extent would you say that your knowledge of health promotion has improved in the past year?" and "To what extent would you say that your skills as a health promotion practitioner have improved in the past year?" In both of our surveys, nearly half of the respondents indicated that their knowledge and skills had improved "a moderate amount" (3 on a 5-point scale). Averaging the results of the two surveys, 42 percent of the HPCs believed their knowledge had improved by "a great deal" (4 or 5 on a 5-point scale). On the same scale, 29 percent of the HPCs believed their skills had improved by "a great deal" (4 or 5 on a 5-point scale). A large majority of HPCs believed that their knowledge and skills had improved by at least a moderate amount. This self-assessed change is substantiated by the ability of virtually all the HPCs to identify specific domains in which their knowledge and skills had improved. During interviews conducted in early 2002, the HPCs identified the following areas of improvement to their knowledge of health promotion and its practice:

- the connections between population health, acute care, and other sectors of activity
- the difficulty of health promotion practice
- the determinants of health
- a more encompassing definition of health
- the various agencies involved in health promotion work
- a range of health promotion strategies, such as community development and the development of supportive public policies
- discrete health issues, such as tobacco, physical activity, and diabetes
- the time required to achieve health promotion results
- the ability to explain health promotion to others
- an appreciation for the multiplicity of skills required to practise population health promotion
- the importance of relationship building and participatory practice
- strategic planning and the use of program logic models
- awareness of sources of funding and other resources for health promotion.

Increases in knowledge tended to be more dramatic for relatively inexperienced practitioners. Those with more previous experience reported greater depth of understanding over time, and a greater level of comfort with their previously existing knowledge.

During the same interviews, the HPCs identified the following areas of improvement in their skills:

- communication skills, including creating displays, writing for the media, making presentations, and using new information technologies
- community development
- nurturing partnerships
- program planning skills, including needs assessment and evaluation

- analyzing the root causes of health outcomes
- assessing the rationale and potential impact of health promotion actions
- being strategic and selective in one's practice
- assessing resources for use in health promotion practice
- providing guidance to others in the understanding and implementation of health promotion
- advocating for health promotion, both within the health district and with the public
- research skills

While we did not ask the HPCs to rate their overall sense of change in their commitment related to health promotion practice, they offered numerous qualitative observations about how such commitment had changed. Briefly, the major changes to the commitment of the health promotion practitioners with whom we worked included:

- coming to a deep, personal understanding of health and health promotion
- embracing socio-environmental models of health promotion
- delegating authority and sharing power
- being more comfortable working behind the scenes instead of generating publicity or statistical indicators of participation in programs
- focusing health promotion efforts on "tougher" issues (such as influencing the "upstream" determinants of health) and more challenging strategies (such as advocacy and policy development)
- working intersectorally and developing important partnerships
- building the capacity of other health district staff
- being strategic in looking for promising avenues for health promotion work
- measuring success in more sophisticated ways than simply counting participants
- positioning themselves and their actions in a stronger community context

Despite having identified important changes to their knowledge, skills, and commitment regarding health promotion, the HPCs, on average, believed that their overall health promotion capacity had improved only modestly during the years preceding our surveys in 2000 and 2001. Averaging the results of the two surveys, one-third of the HPCs viewed their overall capacity as "relatively unchanged," while 44 percent viewed their capacity as "somewhat better" and only 10 percent viewed their capacity as "much better." About 13 percent of the HPCs perceived a decline in their capacity over time.

There is an apparent gap between the HPCs' self-assessed progress in terms of their knowledge, skills, and commitment with regard to health promotion and their overall sense of the development of their capacity. This gap was understood, by the HPCs, as a reflection of the resources available to them to engage in health promotion work. In 2000 and 2001, we asked the HPCs to rate the importance of seventeen resources to their health promotion practice, and to assess whether their access to those resources had declined or increased in the year preceding the survey. Table 5.1 shows the results of these questions.

The left-hand columns of Table 5.1 simply rank (on a five-point scale) the HPCs' views of different resources as having a strong influence on their practice. The relative ranking of the different resources can be seen from the table. Resources very close to the HPCs (e.g., their own energy, time, and other responsibilities; the support and understanding of their managers) were consistently rated highly. Public and non-district practitioner support and understanding were rated as less important, as was access to computers, the Internet, and program materials or kits.

The right-hand columns of Table 5.1 can be understood by looking at a score of 2.0 as meaning that the resource in question, on average for the HPCs as a group, stayed the same over the year preceding the date of the survey. Means lower than two imply that the availability of the resource (in the view of the HPCs) declined. In both years, the resource that was in the steepest decline was the time available to do health promotion work. Ironically, none of the resources that were improving the most (e.g., Internet and computer access, and support from non-district practitioners) were among the resources rated as being most important to health promotion practice. Comparing the results in 2001 with those of the year 2000, there were a few notable shifts in the HPCs' views of how their resources were changing. Whereas in 2000 the HPCs had replied that management and board support and understanding were declining, in 2001 the HPCs replied that such understanding and support were increasing. Whereas in 2000 the HPCs had replied that public understanding and their own personal energy and enthusiasm were increasing, in 2001 the HPCs replied that such resources were declining.

Conclusions

Individual capacity for health promotion is a concept that refers to the

Table 5.1

Influence of resources on practice

Resources[a]	Strength of influence on practice[b]		Change in resource in past year[c]	
	2000	2001	2000	2001
Personal energy and enthusiasm	4.24	4.46	2.14	1.96
Management understanding of HP[d]	4.24	4.35	1.86	2.13
Conflicting workload responsibilities	4.20	4.15	2.41	2.54
Management support for HP	4.20	4.38	1.73	2.13
Staff resources dedicated to HP	4.17	4.35	1.68	1.83
District colleagues' support for HP	4.12	4.35	2.09	2.04
Time available to do HP	4.08	4.35	1.62	1.71
Financial resources dedicated to HP	4.04	4.15	1.81	1.79
District colleagues' HP understanding	3.96	4.31	2.18	2.13
Board support for HP	3.92	4.19	1.77	2.08
Board understanding of HP	3.88	4.19	1.91	2.04
Easy access to a computer at work	3.88	4.31	2.33	2.13
Easy access to the Internet at work	3.76	4.27	2.29	2.21
Easy access to program materials/kits	3.76	3.92	2.18	2.08
Public support for HP	3.68	3.96	1.86	1.88
Public understanding of HP	3.52	4.04	2.14	1.96
Support from HP practitioners outside the district	3.52	3.56	2.32	2.21

a N varies from 21 to 26.
b Influence of resources on practice was measured on a 5-point scale, with 1 = "not at all" and 5 = "a great deal."
c Change in resource over the past year was measured on a 3-point scale, with 1 = "decreased," 2 = "stayed the same," and 3 = "increased."
d HP = health promotion.

knowledge, skills, commitment, and resources that enable practitioners to engage in effective health promotion activities. The first section of this chapter described the key elements of individual capacity. The second section examined the process of capacity development in relatively abstract terms, while the third described the process of capacity development in terms of the concrete experiences of the practitioners with whom we worked during the BHPC project. In summary, while the process of individual capacity building could logically be deduced from the elements of capacity defined in Figure 5.1, in practice the evolution of capacity among practitioners depended on certain key catalysts: (1) having the support of managers and colleagues; (2) assuming new professional roles or responsibilities; (3) encountering new ideas and practices through such means as continuing education, networking, and resource materials; and (4) practising newly acquired knowledge and skills in significant projects and partnerships.

One of our most interesting conclusions is that building the capacity of individual practitioners has only a limited influence on improving health promotion practice. There is no doubt that processes such as continuing education, networking, and staff development are important for the development of the knowledge, skills, and commitment of individual practitioners. In Chapter 4 we documented how individual practitioners learned and changed their health promotion practices through our continuing education and networking interventions. In this chapter we demonstrated how the capacity of individual health promotion practitioners evolves. However, the ability of those individual practitioners to act in the world is influenced by factors that transcend their individual capacities. The organizational context within which they work and the larger environment within which their organization is situated have a substantial impact on the ability of health promotion practitioners to realize their capacity and put it into action.

There is a parallel between the development of individual capacity for health promotion work and the efforts of individual practitioners to influence the health of the populations with which they work. Just as there are limits to the effectiveness of individualized approaches to health promotion, so there are limits to capacity-building approaches that focus on the individual practitioner. In health promotion, other things being equal, it is important that individuals make healthy lifestyle choices. In capacity development for health promotion practice, other things being equal, it is important that practitioners have high levels of knowledge, skills, and commitment. However, in capacity development just as in health promotion, "other things" are never equal. In health promotion, the social and material environment within which individuals live has a profound influence on their behaviours and health status. In capacity development, organizational and environmental factors have a substantial influence on the capacities and actions of individual practitioners.

Developing the capacity of individual practitioners is essential to accomplishing more effective health promotion work, but it is not sufficient on its own. Without organizational development and environmental change, efforts to develop the capacities of individual practitioners may lead to yet another parallel with individualized approaches to health promotion: blaming the victim. Effective health promotion practice requires effective health promotion practitioners. However, as we will show in the next two chapters, effective health promotion practice also requires organizational and environmental settings that foster and support such practice. The most capacity-rich practitioner cannot work effectively on his or her own; implying that this is possible through capacity development strategies that focus exclusively on practitioners is unfair to the practitioners. Just as individuals may internalize the social problems at the root of their individual health outcomes, so practitioners may internalize the sense of inadequacy or failure that comes from practising health promotion in an environment that inhibits effective practice.

6
Organizations

The capacity of organizations must be understood quite differently from that of individuals. While not wishing to derail our narrative of health promotion capacity building with an extended ontological debate, we must emphasize that organizations cannot "have capacity" in the same manner as individuals, because organizations do not exist in the same way that individuals do. Organizations are not entities that may be said to exist in the way that individual human beings, by virtue of their physiological nature, exist. Rather, organizations are constructed and maintained by individuals, through relationships with other individuals. Organizations exist as patterns of relationships between people. These patterns of relationships include interactions between people, and the ideas with which people make sense of such interactions. Organizations come to be perceived as "things" because patterns of relationships between human beings become regular over time, and because these regularities become structured by written texts (e.g., policy documents and strategic plans) and constructed physical spaces (e.g., buildings and offices). Despite these regularities and the resulting appearance of an objective existence, organizations are always works in progress, socially constructed through the interactions of human beings.

It is absurd to suggest that organizations possess knowledge, skills, or commitment in the same manner that individuals do. However, it does not follow that organizational capacity to engage in health promotion activities can be only the sum of the capacities of the individuals who constitute that organization. Rather, certain patterns of relationships are more likely than others to enable members of an organization to have an impact on the world beyond the boundaries of that organization. Organizational capacity refers to those patterns of relationships that enable members of organizations to effectively engage in health promotion activities.

Organizations, strictly speaking, cannot "act." However, organizations structure patterns of relationships that make certain actions (on the part of individuals) more or less likely. Organizations facilitate certain actions and hinder others. In health promotion, organizations facilitate effective practices through at least the following roles: (1) motivating practitioners by giving them a larger sense of purpose and direction; (2) rewarding practitioners for their actions and expressing pride in their accomplishments; (3) helping practitioners continue to develop their individual capacity, both through formal professional development opportunities and through support of innovative practice and experiential learning; (4) enabling practitioners to gain synergies and learn from working with others; (5) facilitating practitioners' access to resources; and (6) paying practitioners' salaries.

In this chapter, we present what we learned about organizational capacity for health promotion among health districts in Saskatchewan. We describe what we learned according to two guiding questions:

- What are the elements that constitute the capacity of organizations to foster and support effective health promotion action?
- How does such capacity develop over time?

The Nature of Health Promotion Capacity at the Organizational Level

Organizational capacity to foster and support effective health promotion practice is composed of commitment, culture, structures, and resources. Figure 6.1 indicates the main elements of health promotion capacity that we have identified as important for organizations.

Commitment

The existence of people, funding, and infrastructure is not enough to foster effective health promotion practice within organizations. People and resources need to be mobilized in a coherent direction, through a shared commitment to achieving certain ends. Health promotion must be valued at all levels of the organization. If only a few, marginalized practitioners value health promotion, then the chances are that an organization will not really foster widespread and effective health promotion action. If, on the other hand, leaders, managers, and employees from all units in the organization consistently understand and value health promotion, then an organization is more likely to foster effective health promotion action.

Figure 6.1

The basic elements of organizational health promotion capacity

Category	Basic elements of capacity
Commitment	• Health promotion is valued at all levels of the organization.
	• There are a shared vision, a mission, and strategies for engaging in population health promotion to address the determinants of health.
	• Walking the talk: policies, programs, and practices are consistent with the organization's vision, mission, and strategies.
	• Partnerships are valued and nurtured both across the organization and with diverse external organizations and communities.
Culture	• Styles of leadership and management empower health promotion practice, foster lifelong learning, and support healthy working environments.
	• Positive and nurturing relationships are fostered among employees.
	• Communication is open and timely, enabling employees to solve problems, learn from mistakes, and share successes.
	• Critical reflection, innovation, and learning are fostered.
Structures	• Health promotion is a shared responsibility, being an integral part of job titles, job descriptions, and performance evaluations among at least several employees.
	• There are effective policies and practices of human resource recruitment, retention, and professional development.
	• There are participatory, empowering, and evidence-based practices for strategic planning, needs assessment, program planning, and evaluation.
	• Employees are organized into work teams that promote intra-institutional collaboration.
Resources	• A significant number of employees in key positions and units have high levels of individual capacity for health promotion.
	• Adequate funding is provided for the programmatic and infrastructural costs of engaging in health promotion activities.
	• Appropriate infrastructure exists, including office space, capital equipment, technology, and effective means of communication.
	• Active engagement with communities brings additional resources.

Commitment should be fostered through both top-down and bottom-up processes. Health promotion should be central to the agenda of the board or other such governance structures, and should be integrated throughout the organization's strategic plan. Organizational leaders and managers should consistently express their commitment to health promotion, and should enable diverse practitioners, at all levels of the organization, to participate in setting the goals and strategies through which this commitment will be operationalized. These participatory processes should lead to concrete statements of shared vision, mission, goals, and strategies for population health promotion. Such statements need to be linked with action through policies and practices that encourage key members of the organization to "walk the talk" of population health promotion. Since influencing the determinants of health is a big job (beyond the realistic capacity of any single practitioner or organization), partnerships must be valued and nurtured both across the organization and with diverse external organizations and communities.

People, resources, and good intentions do not necessarily translate into effective health promotion actions. Effective action will be facilitated if the culture and structures that characterize relationships within an organization support such action. Organizational culture refers to those aspects of relationships in organizations that characterize the nature of individuals' day-to-day activities. Organizational structures refer to aspects of relationships in organizations that are written down, and institutionalized to the extent that they transcend the day-to-day activities of individuals in the organization. Commitment to health promotion is an important starting point for the development of effective culture and structures.

Culture

Figure 6.1 identifies four elements of organizational culture that enable individuals within organizations to more effectively practice health promotion. Styles of leadership and management must empower health promotion practice, foster lifelong learning, and support healthy working environments. Leaders of organizations have important responsibilities for facilitating an organizational culture within which health promotion practice can flourish. Leadership development is an enormous industry, and huge numbers of books have been written about effective leadership styles and practices. We have learned that leaders of organizations can make a difference to the capacity of individuals within those organizations to undertake health promotion work. Leadership for health promotion involves both serving as a champion for the health promotion cause and being able to mobilize people to contribute to shared health promotion goals. Effective leaders understand the big health promotion picture and have an empowering leadership style.

Positive and nurturing relationships must be fostered among employees at all levels and in all units. Obviously, negative interpersonal relationships in any organization deflect the energy and focus of employees from accomplishing the goals toward which they would otherwise strive. Positive and nurturing relationships facilitate the development of capacity by all individuals involved in such relationships. The maintenance of positive and nurturing relationships in an organization involves ongoing processes for problem solving and conflict resolution. Communication must be open and timely, enabling employees to solve problems, learn from mistakes, and share successes. Good leadership, positive interpersonal relationships, and healthy patterns of communication all encourage critical reflection, innovation, and learning.

Structures
Organizational capacity for health promotion is enhanced when health promotion is structurally defined as a shared responsibility. Such structural definition can be operationalized in job titles and job descriptions, and integrated into performance appraisals and reporting or accountability mechanisms. A marker of organizational capacity is when one person is designated to be responsible for health promotion, fulfilling a leadership and coordination role. This individual serves as a link for other staff and the public, and educates others about health promotion. The designation of a key health promotion point person is necessary yet insufficient for organizational capacity. One designated individual cannot single-handedly increase organizational health promotion capacity. To be sufficient, health promotion needs to be a shared responsibility among many staff. Increasing a sense of shared ownership of organizational capacity for health promotion involves encouraging all staff to increase their understanding of health promotion. All staff should seek opportunities to incorporate health promotion principles in their area of work. Appropriate structures facilitate collaborative action. This can be accomplished through the establishment of a health promotion unit or team, multidisciplinary teams for addressing issues of shared interest, and health promotion committees with representation from various levels within the organization. Health promotion teams or committees can include representatives from other organizations.

Since human resources are a prerequisite to health promotion action, organizational capacity for health promotion is enhanced when effective policies and practices are in place to recruit, retain, and improve the capacities of practitioners. The recruitment and retention of good employees is not particularly different in the field of health promotion than elsewhere. Apart from instrumental reasons, people are attracted to jobs and stay in them because they find the work challenging and meaningful, they like the people with whom they work, and they feel respected and appreciated. A sense of ownership and autonomy with regard to one's work is an important motivation. Such motivation can be fostered through organizational structures that are reasonably egalitarian and enable practitioners to participate in decisions about work assignments.

Recruiting and retaining good people is one side of the human resource challenge to organizational capacity in health promotion. Enhancing the capacity of such people is the other side. Individual capacity for health promotion is described thoroughly in Chapter 5. However, organizations have a role in facilitating the ongoing development of practitioners' capacity. Building the capacity of staff involves supporting professional development through at least the following major strategies: (1) participation in formal continuing education; (2) engagement in formal and informal networks; (3) opportunities to innovate, experiment, take risks, and learn from mistakes in one's professional practice; and (4) time and support for critical reflection on one's practice.

Each of these strategies involves the investment of time on the part of practitioners, and most involve some expenditure of other resources on the part of the organization. Structural encouragement to consistently make such investments is an important element of organizational capacity for health promotion.

Organizational capacity for health promotion involves creating structural frameworks within which competent individuals will consider their job to be about health promotion, know how to do that job, and be motivated to do it well. One challenge of organizational structure is to institutionalize certain key processes so that their accomplishment does not depend on the ongoing judgments of individual practitioners. For example, empowering and evidence-based processes for strategic planning, needs assessment, program planning, and evaluation should be institutionalized so that practitioners are compelled to follow best-practice guidelines in these areas. While individuals must be given the latitude to practise health promotion work according to their personal backgrounds and professional judgments, they must not determine why and how to engage in various programs and initiatives based only on intuitive or habitual practices. It is the structural responsibility of organizations to ensure that individual practitioners follow empowering and evidence-based processes in their work.

Organizational capacity for health promotion involves structuring work teams in ways that facilitate rather than impede collaboration within the organization. Effective health promotion practice is difficult when health promotion staff are isolated by organizational barriers or reporting structures, or when responsibilities for health promotion are shared among many staff without effective accountability measures.

Resources

Resources are central to organizational capacity to foster and support health promotion action. Human resources are important. Employees having high levels of individual capacity (see Figure 5.1) are integral to organizational capacity, as is the location of these employees in positions where they have the power to influence the actions of others. Financial and infrastructural resources are also important. Funding can be made available through the core budget of the organization, through external grants and contracts, or through partnerships with external agencies and communities. Key roles of organizations in health promotion work are to facilitate the access of individual practitioners to tools and resources, and to support individual and team development. The ability to dedicate or access financial and infrastructural resources for health promotion is clearly an element of organizational capacity.

Active engagement with community members is a valuable resource for organizational capacity for health promotion. Capitalizing on communities as a resource can be achieved primarily through communication and interaction. Organizations can seek opportunities to hear from the public through such activities as regular communication with specific community groups, health surveys and community profiling, and invitations to participate in public forums. In turn, organizations can seek opportunities to connect with the public by implementing actions to address and meet expressed community needs, regularly advancing community understanding of health promotion through reports and the media, and fostering volunteerism in health promotion initiatives and committees. Through such interactions, both organizational and community capacity for health promotion can be nurtured.

Limits to the Efficacy of Organizational Capacity

Organizations such as the regional health districts with which we worked over the course of BHPC have important roles in health promotion action. Such organizations employ health promotion practitioners and facilitate the access of those practitioners to resources needed to engage in health promotion. Leaders and peers within such organizations motivate and reward practitioners and give them opportunities to become more effective in their work. However, the capacity of organizations to effectively support health promotion activities is constrained by factors over which those organizations have limited control. These factors are determined by the social environment in which the organizations exist. In Chapter 7, we document the environmental influences on health promotion capacity that were most significant for our work in Saskatchewan. At this point, it is important simply to recognize that organizational capacity for health promotion does not translate directly into effective health promotion action. Environmental factors mediate the manner in which capacity is translated into action.

The Development of Organizational Health Promotion Capacity
The capacity of organizations to foster and support effective health promotion action is constituted by the range of elements identified in Figure 6.1. In abstract terms, the development of organizational capacity is a logical process of enhancing the commitment, culture, structures, and resources of the organization so that it is better prepared to support health promotion action. In the real world, however, the linear progression toward greater organizational capacity is very often made complex by the nature of individuals and their organizations. While capacity development should ideally involve the progressive building of greater capacity within each of the elements of capacity we have defined, this was not the experience of the health districts with which we worked. The history of capacity development among these organizations was more complex than some logical progression toward a predetermined goal of greater capacity.

As was the case with the health promotion capacity of individual practitioners, understanding the evolution of any organization's capacity to support health promotion requires attention to the history of the organization. At the same time, there are certain regularities in the seemingly idiosyncratic experiences of organizations that enable us to make generalizations about the kinds of factors and experiences that tend to help or hinder capacity development. Despite the complexity and diversity of the development of health promotion capacity among organizations, it is possible to identify major catalysts to the development of organizational capacity for health promotion. In the experience of the health districts, organization capacity was:

- nurtured by opportunities for individuals and teams to work on meaningful projects and partnerships
- nurtured by access to resources targeted toward health promotion
- nurtured by externally driven planning and evaluation exercises
- nurtured by individual capacity building
- both helped and hindered by changes in key personnel
- both helped and hindered by organizational restructuring
- nurtured by the strategic action of change agents

Each of these claims is briefly discussed below, with illustrations from the health districts.

Organizational capacity was nurtured by opportunities for individuals and teams to work on meaningful projects. Health district staff engaged in a variety of health promotion projects that had the effect of enhancing and disseminating capacity to engage in health promotion. Specific projects included those in the areas of: diabetes prevention, tobacco reduction, youth wellness, food security and nutrition enhancement, school-based activities, parenting and family health, maternal and women's health, early childhood, heart health, physical activity, public awareness or health education, violence and abuse prevention, and sexual health and HIV prevention. Concrete projects enhanced the public profiles of districts, attracted positive public and media attention, encouraged volunteer participation, reached diverse audiences, and built linkages and partnerships. Such projects developed individual capacities, built more effective teams, and enhanced organizational receptivity to health promotion work. In an important sense, actually carrying out health promotion work was a key facilitator of enhancing organizational capacity for further health promotion work.

A particularly important form of "experiential capacity development" by individuals and teams in health districts was working in partnership. Several forms of partnership were important catalysts to the development of organizational capacity for health promotion.

Internal partnerships were formed when individuals and teams from one unit (or discipline) within the health district worked with people from other units (or disciplines). For example, health promotion practitioners found partnerships with clinicians, public health nurses, and mental health workers to be valuable means of engaging in health promotion projects.

Lateral partnerships were formed when individuals and teams from one health district worked with people from other health districts. Such partnerships were seen as means to achieve economies of scale in health promotion work, as well as to promote mutual learning and the sharing of ideas, expertise, and resources. For example, several practitioners cited their collaboration with other districts in diabetes prevention initiatives as a valuable lateral partnership.

Community partnerships were formed when individuals and teams from health districts worked with community leaders and volunteers. Working with community was seen both as a key strategy for engaging in health promotion and as a means of building the capacity of communities to work beyond the limited resources of the health districts.

Intersectoral partnerships were formed when individuals and teams from health districts worked with people in organizations from sectors other than health care. Education, social services, recreation, and justice were frequently identified as sectors from which organizations would partner with health districts on joint initiatives. A significant example of intersectoral partnerships during the course of the BHPC project was the establishment of regional intersectoral committees on human services, in which many health districts participated.

Organizational capacity was nurtured by access to resources targeted toward health promotion. Fiscal constraints were consistently reported as a key barrier to enhanced health promotion capacity among health districts in Saskatchewan. It is not surprising, therefore, that many district leaders considered the acquisition of financial resources as a key catalyst to capacity development. In the health districts with which we worked, financial resources were accessed through a variety of external sources, such as the Rural Health Initiatives Fund and provincial initiatives for tobacco reduction and diabetes prevention.

The nature of financial resources applied to health promotion was a two-sided coin in many health districts. On the positive side, access to ad hoc or programmatic funding made possible the hiring of health promotion practitioners, and gave individuals and teams the experience of running health promotion projects. On the negative side, the fact that substantial "core" health district resources were only rarely invested in health promotion led to an insecurity in staffing arrangements and a marginalization of the status of health promotion compared with other district activities. The reliance of health promotion activities and staff on "soft" money led to difficulties in recruiting and retaining excellent practitioners, and to challenges with sustaining programs and projects. Also, targeted funding was more typically available for shorter-term, disease-specific initiatives than for longer-term community development processes.

In addition to financial resources, health district access to other resources supported organizational capacity for health promotion. One example was Saskatchewan Health's publication in 1999 of *A Population Health Promotion Framework for Saskatchewan Health Districts*. This document introduced the principles, values, and strategies of population health promotion, and was used to educate health district board members and staff. Another example was the distribution by the Saskatchewan Health Population Health Branch (1997) of a resource binder on population health promotion. The binder included copy-ready materials on health determinants, strategies for action, and evidence for the efficacy of population health promotion.

Organizational capacity was nurtured by externally driven planning and evaluation exercises. For example, the Achieving Improved Measures (AIM) accreditation process of the Canadian Council on Health Services Accreditation incorporated population health promotion principles and required the formation of cross-organizational work teams. This accreditation process gave health promotion staff an opportunity to take a leadership role and to provide education about health promotion within the health district. Accreditation increased collective understanding of health promotion, and increased the sense of shared ownership of health promotion responsibilities. In another example, the establishment of health districts was accompanied by a mandatory needs assessment process through which the new districts were required to establish goals and objectives that reflected the conditions and priorities of the populations within the districts. In a third example, each district was required to submit a strategic plan to Saskatchewan Health for 1999-2003. Accreditation, needs assessment, and strategic planning were integral to building commitment to health promotion in many districts, and such processes frequently led to the establishment of organizational structures supportive of health promotion. In some districts, the initial needs assessment process led to the establishment of community initiatives committees, while in others it led to the establishment of community grants programs.

Organizational capacity was nurtured by individual capacity building. Since the nature of individual capacity and its enhancement was discussed in Chapter 5, here we simply observe that individual capacity building may be a key catalyst to broader organizational development. The capacity of an organization is, of course, dependent on the capacity of the individuals whose activities and relationships constitute that organization. Individual capacity may be built through the development of the human resources within an organization or by the recruitment of new people. Organizational commitment to continuing education among a wide range of staff was an important starting point for developing broad-based individual capacity, as was assigning increased roles and responsibilities to capable individuals.

Organizational capacity was both helped and hindered by changes in key personnel. On the one hand, the appointment of a medical health officer, chief executive officer, or other senior manager with strong leadership abilities and a commitment to health promotion led to improvements in capacity across some health districts. The role of leaders as champions for health promotion was important for the development of capacity in several districts. Conversely, the departure of such leaders sometimes led to a decline in capacity. At a more operational level, the ability to recruit and retain capacity-rich health promotion practitioners obviously helped some districts enhance their capacity. In other districts, extended leaves, lack of replacement staff, and an inability to recruit qualified staff deflated health promotion capacity.

Organizational capacity was both helped and hindered by organizational restructuring. The most significant restructuring came in 2002, when the thirty-two health districts were amalgamated by the provincial government into twelve regional health authorities. The impact of this restructuring on the capacity of the organizations in the system to support health promotion work remains to be seen. Earlier and more modest experiences of restructuring in the health districts had varying effects on organizational capacity for health promotion. Fiscal constraint and downsizing frequently led to restructuring in the 1990s. Such restructuring was sometimes seen as positive for health promotion capacity, as it led to decreased emphasis on acute care facilities and an increased commitment to health promotion. In other cases, such restructuring was seen as negative for health promotion capacity, as all available resources and attention were transferred to acute care services and the organizational commitment to health promotion was marginalized by the need to keep the acute care system functioning.

One specific form of organizational restructuring that was a catalyst to capacity development was the establishment of discrete teams dedicated to health promotion. Such restructuring was important in three ways. First, it sometimes enabled the accumulation of human and financial resources that directly facilitated health promotion action. Second, it sometimes placed individuals with high health promotion capacity in structural positions where they could influence organizational commitment and culture with regard to health promotion. Third, it sometimes indicated the recognition of senior managers and the board that health promotion was a significant organizational priority. Thus, for both material and symbolic reasons, the establishment of a health promotion team helped build organizational capacity. For similar reasons, the designation of a health promotion person to a fairly senior management position (e.g., director of health promotion) was often cited as a factor in developing health promotion capacity.

Of course, restructuring and the appointment of staff to formal health promotion positions was a two-sided coin in many health districts. There were three key risks associated with such restructuring. First, just as health promotion capacity was sometimes enhanced by the formation of a work team in the organization, so was such capacity diminished by the dismantling or reduction of such teams. Second, there was a chronic problem, across many health districts, regarding the diverse and often burdensome responsibilities of health promotion staff. Health promotion personnel frequently had to juggle their health promotion work with responsibilities in areas such as clinical services, staff development, and strategic planning. Merely holding a number of different roles was not the problem; indeed, some practitioners commented that having multiple roles enhanced their practice if such roles fit together with an appropriate health promotion focus. Third, formally designating leadership in health promotion to particular individuals and teams created a risk that other people in the health district would then conclude that health promotion was now officially outside their realm of concern.

Organizational capacity was nurtured by the strategic action of change agents. Agents of change were defined both by their personal characteristics and by their structural position within health districts. The personal characteristics of an effective change agent for health promotion included being:

- philosophically committed to, and articulate about, health promotion
- enthusiastic, passionate, and skilled at marketing health promotion
- courageous enough to take risks
- flexible, patient, and persistent
- able to consult, build relationships, and coordinate efforts
- informed, credible, and respected
- knowledgeable about the organization and the community
- a role model of the willingness to change

Having the right personal characteristics was necessary but not sufficient for being an effective change agent for health promotion. Individual efficacy to make change in organizations depended on having the power to influence the thoughts and actions of others. This power sometimes arose from structural positions or mandates (e.g., the CEO or medical health officer as agent of change), and sometimes arose from the organization of people into networks or work teams. The designation of Health Promotion Contacts by each district created the potential for making change through both structural and networked forms of power. In some cases, HPCs had the responsibility, mandate, and skill to educate and coach others in health promotion, to encourage broad participation among staff and the general public, and to evaluate the effectiveness of health promotion activities. In these cases, individual agents of change made substantial contributions to organizational capacity for health promotion.

Conclusions

Organizational capacity for health promotion is a concept that refers to patterns of relationships between people that foster and support effective health promotion activities. The first part of this chapter described the key elements of organizational capacity, within categories defined as commitment, culture, structures, and resources. The second part examined the process of capacity development, and found that the following key factors tended to catalyze the development of organizational capacity: (1) meaningful projects and partnerships, (2) access to resources, (3) externally driven planning and evaluation exercises, (4) individual capacity building, (5) organizational restructuring, and (6) change agents.

The evolution of capacity among health districts in Saskatchewan was not a linear process over the decade of their existence. At different points in time, different districts experienced gains and losses in capacity. Given the fundamental restructuring of the health district system during the course of the BHPC project, we cannot offer an assessment of the actual evolution of organizational capacity in Saskatchewan as we did for individual practitioners in Chapter 5. It is not possible to describe a typical pathway through which districts systematically built capacity. It is possible, however, to describe the common ways in which the environment for health promotion both promoted and constrained the development of capacity among these complex and diverse organizations. In the next chapter, we examine environmental influences on the evolution of individual and organizational capacity for health promotion.

7
The Environment

In Chapters 5 and 6, we argued that there are important interrelationships between the capacity of individuals and organizations to engage in health promotion. We showed how individual practitioners require a supportive organizational framework within which to work, and how organizational capacity to provide such a framework is determined by the nature of relationships between individuals. Further, we argued that external factors constrain, promote, and mediate the health promotion capacity of individuals and organizations. As a set, such factors may be conceptualized as the environment for health promotion capacity. In this chapter, we explore the manner in which environmental variables influence health promotion capacity.

As we did when introducing the concept of organizational capacity for health promotion, we begin this chapter with a brief caution against reifying the concept of "environment." Of course, the environment has very real implications for the thoughts and actions of human beings. We are all, to some extent, prisoners of the material and symbolic worlds that we inherit from previous generations. However, the environment should not be understood as some universal and monolithic entity, beyond the capacity of individual human beings to reproduce or challenge. In fact, the environment is constantly in flux: it is produced, sustained, and changed through the actions of a multitude of individuals. Human environments tend to be relatively stable, since the actions of individuals are rooted in those individuals' prior experiences of the world, and such experiences reflect, of course, an existing environment. Despite appearances, however, the environment is not immutable, nor does it stand outside the realm of human interaction. That is why, in this chapter focusing on the influence that environments have on the health promotion capacity of individuals and organizations, our conclusions explore the ways in which individuals and organizations may influence the environment for health promotion.

We described the social context for health promotion capacity in Saskatchewan in Chapter 2. That chapter examined the social changes that characterized the province in the latter part of the twentieth century, the public policy frameworks within which the health care sector evolved in the 1990s, and the administrative and legal arrangements that characterized the rise and fall of the health district system from the early 1990s to the early years of the twenty-first century. Against the backdrop of this overall context, we now explore the key environmental variables influencing the health promotion capacity of individuals and organizations.

The Nature of the Environment for Health Promotion

At one level, understanding the environment for health promotion is as complex and daunting as unravelling the mysteries of the universe. The practice of health promotion in Saskatchewan is one small part of a great big world characterized by complex and shifting social, economic, political, cultural, and natural realities. Understanding the environment for health promotion means knowing something about these realities, and how they are experienced and produced by people far from Saskatchewan. At another level, however, it is possible to identify a relatively small number of key influences that provide the most immediate context for health promotion practice in Saskatchewan. While it is important to recognize that these immediate influences are themselves determined by far more complex local, regional, national, and global processes, it is useful to understand these immediate influences in their own right. We argue that key environmental variables influencing the health promotion capacity of individuals and organizations include political will, public opinion, the existence of supportive organizations, and the availability of ideas and other resources.

Political Will

The health promotion capacity of the individuals and organizations we worked with was closely linked to the status of health districts as quasi-governmental organizations. The existence, structure, mandate, and financing of the health districts were dependent on processes of forming and operating governments in Saskatchewan. The dependency of these organizations on political processes strongly influenced the ability of health districts to undertake health promotion work, and eventually led to their major restructuring as organizational entities. Three key processes were at work. First, overall levels of funding for the health districts were set by the allocation of tax revenues. Given Canadian economic realities in recent years, this means that fiscal constraint was a nearly constant driving force. The political will to devote resources to the health district system was constrained by competing priorities for the fiscal resources of the provincial government.

Second, investment of health district financial and human resources in health promotion activities was challenged by the districts' mandate to engage in clinical services and acute care. Political will to invest in health promotion in addition to other health system priorities was variable at two levels. At the provincial level, Saskatchewan Health encouraged investment in health promotion and prevention by providing core funding with a "one-way valve" that enabled health districts to transfer funding from acute care services to community programs (including health promotion and prevention) but not in the other direction. Because of pressure from the acute care sector, however, Saskatchewan Health was ultimately reluctant to enforce the one-way valve provisions of its core funding. Although Saskatchewan Health never dedicated core funding expressly to population health promotion, the Rural Health Initiatives Fund did allocate funding to health promotion and prevention initiatives. The relatively small proportion of core funding mandated for prevention and public health, compared with the amounts dedicated to acute and long-term care services, marginalized the practice of health promotion both symbolically and materially. At the health district level, leaders and managers had to allocate scarce resources among the various mandates of their organizations. Such resource allocation decisions depended not simply on the rational calculation of the impact of different investments on the health outcomes of the population but also on the political realities of leading quasi-governmental organizations.

Third, local and provincial political will to invest in health promotion was eroded by ongoing public (or at least media) fixation on hospital closures and other acute care issues. The political will to invest in health promotion was often weakened because decision makers worried about the electoral and other consequences of any public perception of erosion of the acute care system. Despite the evidence and logic behind investing resources in health promotion, it was difficult for elected officials and their appointed representatives to ignore agitation with regard to things like funding for medications, surgical waiting lists, and emergency room congestion. Funding for prevention and health promotion was deferred until acute care problems could be resolved.

Public Opinion

Political will to support health promotion activities was influenced by public opinion. Here, the basic context introduced in Chapter 2 was very important. Health districts in Saskatchewan were formed at the same time that a "wellness" approach to health care was adopted by the provincial government, which also coincided with the introduction of substantial fiscal restraint, including the closure of fifty-two small hospitals in the province. As such, the idea of health promotion constantly struggled to overcome the public perception that the "wellness" agenda was merely an excuse for the government to spend less money on health care services. Through the 1990s, media attention was frequently given to a range of concerns in the health care system, including surgical waiting lists, lack of physicians in rural areas, lack of specialists in urban areas, labour relations crises among various professional groups, and a pervading sense of malaise about the funding and quality of medical care in the province. Due to the timing of its adoption by the provincial government, the "wellness" agenda and, by implication, health promotion became associated in the minds of some people with the closure of hospitals, the reduction of health care staff, and the loss of services.

Many health promotion practitioners and leaders believed that public opinion regarding acute care services was a key environmental challenge to the development of health promotion capacity in Saskatchewan. They believed that public opinion made it difficult for the provincial government to direct additional resources toward population health promotion, and for health district boards to give priority to health promotion. While concerns about the acute care system were one problematic aspect of public opinion, another was the lack of understanding about health promotion beyond lifestyle change and health education.

Population health promotion is an approach to health promotion that poses some challenges to traditional approaches such as individual health education and mass media messages about the importance of personal lifestyle change. Important as those are, they do not address the environmental conditions that constrain individual choices, and they do not take into account policies and community contexts having a less direct but equally important influence on individual decisions and individual health status. Even though many people understand the importance of such socio-environmental determinants, many others continue to regard action on such determinants as outside the mandate of the health system. Health is, for many, intimately associated with health "care" and associated medical services. To many, promoting health means eating well and getting enough exercise to avoid disease. From this point of view, efforts in population health promotion to encourage action beyond these immediate concerns are at best puzzling and at worst a threat to the investment of energy and resources in "real" health system issues. Limited understanding of population health promotion also exists among health professionals. Initial training typically does not equip practitioners to work comfortably in approaches such as community development and the empowerment of action by lay people and communities.

Supportive Organizations

While political will and public opinion were widely considered to be constraints to the development of health promotion capacity in Saskatchewan, the existence of supportive organizations was considered to be of substantial benefit to such capacity. This benefit was experienced in two ways. First, many organizations, both within and outside the health care sector, took direct action on the determinants of health. Within the sector, many organizations were recognized by health promotion leaders as contributing to an environment supportive of health promotion capacity. These included groups and associations of health practitioners, including the District Health Promotion Contacts Group and the Saskatchewan Public Health Association (SPHA); the Saskatchewan Association of Health Organizations (SAHO); research organizations such as the Health Services Utilization and Research Commission (HSURC) and the Saskatchewan Population Health Evaluation and Research Unit (SPHERU); and disease-specific organizations such as the Heart and Stroke Foundation of Saskatchewan, the Cancer Society, and the Canadian Diabetes Association. Outside the health sector, action on determinants was taken by school divisions, municipalities, community social development agencies, faith communities, and recreation groups, among others.

Second, various forms of collaboration among organizations enabled health promotion practitioners with the health districts to work more effectively. The various forms of partnership in which health districts participated were described in the previous chapter. However, the existence of supportive province-wide organizations was an important feature of the environment for health promotion because such organizations provided: (1) direct partnerships in health promotion programs and initiatives; (2) financial, logistical, and staffing support for health promotion programs and initiatives; (3) colleagues and other sources of learning and support with regard to health promotion practice; and (4) a sense of purpose to practitioners who might otherwise have perceived themselves as isolated individuals struggling with issues beyond their realistic capacity to influence.

The contribution of intersectoral partnerships to health promotion was facilitated by the existence of several significant initiatives whose primary mandates were to encourage synergies between individuals and organizations working in different sectors. An example unique to Saskatchewan was the Saskatchewan Population Health Promotion Partnership (SPHPP), formed in 1996 to support and strengthen population health promotion in Saskatchewan (see Chapter 4). Another unique Saskatchewan partnership was the Human Services Integration Forum (HSIF), with Regional Intersectoral Committees (RICs) throughout the province. These committees demonstrated provincial government commitment to working intersectorally and provided opportunities for health districts to partner with other sectors to work on determinants such as literacy, job-readiness, youth development, and poverty. HSIF used a population health promotion model as its framework for action. The semi-annual forums sponsored by HSIF facilitated discussion of issues related to community development and the population health promotion model. Several major HSIF initiatives provided policy frameworks for action, including a Child Action Plan and an Early Childhood Policy Framework.

While the existence of supportive organizations was, overall, a benefit to the development of health promotion capacity in Saskatchewan from 1998 to 2003, the role of governments seemed to have both positive and negative outcomes. As discussed above, sustaining the political will to invest public resources in the health promotion activities of health districts was a consistent challenge. From the perspective of many practitioners and leaders within the health districts, the provincial government at a political level did not provide consistent and supportive leadership for the health promotion agenda. While early health reform initiatives emphasized the importance of health promotion, this commitment was perceived to have evaporated over time, with an increasing emphasis on solving acute care crises and budget deficits.

Ideas and Other Resources
The existence of supportive organizations was one example of how resources from the environment influenced the health promotion capacity of individuals and organizations. Another key resource was the existence of ideas that health promotion practitioners could assess, adapt, and apply to their practice. Such ideas could be placed on a continuum, with general principles at one end and program kits at the other end. In

between, useful ideas about how to engage in health promotion could take a variety of forms, including tools, frameworks, conceptualizations, and program planning materials. The federal and provincial governments offered many programs that provided ideas (and often support funding) for taking health promotion action. Key publications included those from the Federal, Provincial, and Territorial Advisory Committee on Population Health (1994, 1999), Health Canada (1998), and Saskatchewan Health, Population Health Branch (1997, 1999). Key national programs included Health Canada's Population Health Fund, the Canadian Diabetes Strategy, and the establishment, within the Canadian Institutes of Health Research, of the Institute of Population and Public Health and the Canadian Population Health Institute. Key provincial programs included the Population Health Promotion Demonstration Projects, Provincial Wellness Grants, and the Rural Health Initiatives Fund.

Federal and provincial governments had important leadership roles in creating an environment for health promotion. There were three key elements of leadership from Health Canada and Saskatchewan Health: legal, intellectual, and resource-based. The provincial government had constitutional jurisdiction for setting the legal parameters of the health care system in Saskatchewan. The development and enforcement of the Health District Act was the main example of legal leadership during the course of the Building Health Promotion Capacity (BHPC) project. The act mandated the health districts to take action on the health status of their populations. To enforce the act, Saskatchewan Health required health districts to engage in strategic planning. To enhance the focus of the health districts on health promotion, Saskatchewan Health asked each district to name a Health Promotion Contact to facilitate liaison with regard to health promotion across the districts.

In addition to setting the legal and financial framework for the health care system, the federal and provincial governments provided intellectual leadership to the work of that system. Over the course of BHPC, each government sponsored a major review of the health care system. In Saskatchewan, the (Fyke) Commission on Medicare was asked to identify key challenges in reforming and improving medicare, ensuring that it remained sustainable and consistent with core values. This commission addressed the need for continued population health promotion efforts in the interests of fairness so that all citizens had an equal chance at good health. The commission (2001, 41) stated: "While the comparatively low cost and large benefit of public health and population strategies are well recognized, the focus of the past 50 years on personal health services and the immediacy of treatment issues has made providing the investments needed for long term health and sustainability of the system more difficult. Without an enhanced focus on these upstream efforts, the strong foundation of health on which treatments can be effective and affordable is lost."

At a national level, the (Romanow) Commission on the Future of Health Care in Canada (2002) was charged with undertaking a dialogue about the future of the Canadian health system and recommending policies that would strike an appropriate balance between investments in prevention and health maintenance and those directed to care and treatment. This report focused largely on personal health services and those currently covered under medicare rather than the public health system and population-based issues.

As mentioned above, each government produced a significant number of publications and policy documents outlining the role of health promotion in the health care system. These documents served as important resources for health promotion practitioners. The preparation of documents and policy statements was also an opportunity to promote health promotion among professional groups, interest groups, and the general public. Provincial and federal governments each provided resources and capacity development support services to the health care system. A range of programs and services in support of health promotion practice was provided by Health Canada's Population and Public Health Branch, as well as by Saskatchewan Health's Population Health Branch. The fact that Health Canada and Saskatchewan Health employed research and program staff in the fields of population health made these two organizations important sources of support for the development of capacity among individuals and organizations in Saskatchewan.

Two distinct environmental resources that supported the development and dissemination of ideas useful to health promotion practitioners were networks and continuing education opportunities. Since continuing education and networking were such an important part of previous chapters, we merely want to state that opportunities for professional development and contact with peers are components of an environment conducive to the development of health promotion capacity. Networks of scholars and practitioners of health promotion are an important resource. The existence of such networks enables practitioners to find resources, test ideas, ask for advice, seek support, and validate their own capacities by contributing to the resolution of other practitioners' challenges. The existence of appropriate continuing education events enables practitioners to encounter new ideas, practise new skills, and build their networks. Chapter 4 described the networking and continuing education initiatives that we organized through BHPC. During the same time that we were active, a substantial number of continuing education initiatives were developed by other organizations.

Conclusions: Influencing the Environment

We have argued that the environment has an important influence on the health promotion capacity of individuals and organizations. In this chapter, we have described how political will, public opinion, the existence of supportive organizations, and the availability of ideas and other resources may facilitate or constrain the capacity of individuals and organizations to engage in health promotion action. Virtually by definition, the environment for health promotion is something beyond the direct control of individual practitioners or the organizations for whom they work. However, individuals and organizations may have an important influence on the environment. As indicated in the introduction to this chapter, the environment is not only a force that constrains the thoughts and actions of human beings but is also in part the product of those thoughts and actions. Although we did not set out to examine the processes through which individuals and organizations may influence the environment, our work with practitioners and health districts gave us some insights into such processes. Briefly, such processes include:

- advocacy, through which individuals and organizations may influence the development of policies and programs by governments and other organizations
- political action, through which individuals and organizations may influence both public opinion and the political will of elected and appointed officials
- engagement with social movements, through which individuals and organizations may influence the underlying structures behind some of the major environmental factors influencing health promotion capacity
- capacity building, through which individuals and organizations may strengthen the abilities of other organizations to support action on the determinants of health
- research and the dissemination of evidence regarding health promotion, through which individuals and organizations may influence the availability of ideas and other resources for subsequent practice

Clearly, there are complex interrelationships between the nature of the environment, the capacity of organizations to foster and support health promotion practice, and the capacity of individuals to engage in such practice. Excellent professional practices flourish in organizational and environmental settings that provide encouragement and resources for such practices. Health-promoting organizations flourish when composed of highly competent individuals and when they exist in an environment conducive to health promotion work. Environments both constrain and nurture opportunities for health promotion work. With strategic action and time, however, environments themselves may be shaped in order to better support the organization and practice of health promotion.

Part 4
Conclusions

8
Reflections on Building Health Promotion Capacity

Action for Learning

Through the Building Health Promotion Capacity (BHPC) project, we learned how to take action for learning through intervention and research. We learned about facilitating the development of capacity among health promotion practitioners and organizations. We learned how to have a substantial, positive impact on a group of practitioners through a carefully designed and executed program of continuing education and networking. Such a program of intervention must engage its stakeholders in participatory processes throughout the program planning cycle, both to ensure that the program is highly valued and to enable such stakeholders to more independently address their own priorities in the future. Such a program of intervention must use exemplary teaching and learning methods, both to maximize the impact of the time invested by participants in continuing education events and to model the process of capacity building. We learned that there are limits to capacity development strategies focusing on the continuing education and networking of individual practitioners, and to those focusing on the development of organizations. Individuals have difficulty translating their capacity into effective action when they work in organizational or environmental contexts that do not support health promotion practice. Organizations in the public sector are subject to public and political pressures that may constrain their capacity to effectively foster and support such practice.

We learned about studying the process of building capacity for health promotion. We learned that research in this field must be based on a sustained engagement with those whose capacity is being studied. Engagement is important because capacity is such a complex phenomenon that it cannot be easily understood based on observations alone, or on superficial efforts to elicit self-assessments from respondents. Sustaining that engagement is important because the type of critical reflection needed to come to an understanding of capacity and its development cannot be generated in a one-time interaction. We have confidence in our findings about the nature of health promotion capacity and its development because those findings emerged and were revised and validated through a five-year dialogue with the practitioners whose capacity we studied. We learned that research in this field cannot rely exclusively on quantitative methods, or even on positivistic assumptions about the nature of social life. Capacity is a concept that is imbued with meaning by those who possess it as well as by those who purport to study it. In order to understand capacity, researchers must employ methods that enable them to interpret the meanings held by participants in their research, and engage in dialogue with those participants and other researchers about the validity and utility of such interpretations.

We also learned that intervention and research are mutually supportive aspects of a coherent approach to building capacity in health promotion. Research practices provide a foundation on which to construct educational and organizational development interventions. Research processes offer unique learning opportunities to the practitioners and leaders whose capacity is being studied. The design, delivery, and evaluation of practical interventions provide a rich source of data and insight for the study of capacity development. When researchers and continuing education practitioners work closely together, learning from intervention and research contributes to both forms of practice.

Learning from Action

From the action we took over the course of the BHPC project, we learned about the nature of health promotion capacity and the manner in which such capacity develops over time. We conceptualized capacity as a set of characteristics or qualities required by individuals and organizations to effectively plan, implement, and evaluate health promotion activities. Individual and organizational capacity to engage in health promotion are interrelated, and are mediated by a range of environmental influences. For individual practitioners, capacity involves elements of knowledge, skill, commitment, and resources. Practitioners need to understand the issues influencing the health of citizens and communities, and to possess the skills and personal commitment needed to implement strategies to address such issues. Individual practitioners apply their capacity for action in the context of the organizations within which they work. The capacity of these organizations, in turn, is determined in part by the knowledge, skills, and commitment of the individuals who compose them. At the organizational level, capacity also entails elements of organizational culture, structure, commitment, and resources. Environmental influences that either enhance or constrain health promotion action include political will, public opinion, the existence of supportive organizations, and the availability of ideas and other resources. Figures 8.1 and 8.2 provide "capacity checklists" that summarize the nature of health promotion capacity at the individual and organizational levels. Each checklist provides a series of statements about health promotion capacity and encourages its users to self-assess their, or their organization's, capacity. The checklists were designed as a practical tool to catalyze reflection, discussion, and action in building capacity for health promotion.

While capacity is an attribute of individuals and organizations, the environment in which such individuals and organizations work may be more or less supportive of health promotion action. Figure 8.3 presents a checklist for the characteristics of an environment conducive to the health promotion capacity of individuals and organizations.

Individuals, organizations, and environments are obviously interconnected. The capacity of individuals to act is enabled, constrained, and mediated by their organizational and environmental settings. The capacity of organizations is constituted in great part by the capacity of the individuals whose actions and relationships define that organization. While the environment influences the capacities and actions of individuals and organizations, the environment may also be influenced by those individuals and organizations. Figure 8.4 presents a simple graphic that links individuals, organizations, and environments in a set of concentric circles.

The connections between individuals, organizations, and environments is particularly evident when we examine how the capacity of individuals and organizations evolves over time. The four key catalysts to the development of individual health promotion capacity are: (1) support of management and colleagues; (2) opportunity to undertake new roles and responsibilities; (3) opportunity to encounter new ideas and practices through means such as continuing education, networking, and the availability of resource materials; and (4) opportunity to apply newly encountered knowledge and practise newly acquired skills in significant projects and partnerships. Clearly, all of these catalysts are dependent upon the existence of organizational and environmental settings that support health promotion practice.

Figure 8.1

Individual health promotion capacity checklist

Category

Knowledge	☐ I have a holistic understanding of health and its determinants.
	☐ I understand the fundamental principles of population health promotion.
	☐ I am familiar with a variety of strategies for health promotion.
	☐ I understand the contexts within which different health promotion strategies are effective.
	☐ I am familiar with the conditions, aspirations, and cultures of the populations with which I work.
Skills	☐ I am able to effectively plan, implement, and evaluate health promotion.
	☐ I communicate effectively with diverse audiences, using a variety of means.
	☐ I work well with others, in a range of roles and contexts.
	☐ I systematically gather and use evidence to guide my practice.
	☐ I am able to build the capacity of communities and organizations with which I work.
	☐ I am strategic and selective in my practice.
Commitment	☐ I have energy, enthusiasm, patience, and persistence in my work.
	☐ I value equity, justice, empowerment, participation, and respect for diversity.
	☐ I am flexible, innovative, and willing to take thoughtful risks
	☐ I learn from my experiences and from those of others.
	☐ I am confident in my abilities, and am credible in the eyes of others.
	☐ I believe in and advocate for health promotion.
Resources	☐ I have adequate time to engage in health promotion practice.
	☐ I have tools to aid my practice so that I am not constantly reinventing the wheel.
	☐ I have the infrastructure needed to practise health promotion.
	☐ I have supportive managers, colleagues, and allies with whom to work and learn.
	☐ I can access adequate financial resources for my health promotion practice.

Figure 8.2

Organizational health promotion capacity checklist

Category

Commitment   ☐ We value health promotion at all levels of our organization.
    ☐ We have a clearly defined vision and mission to engage in health promotion.
    ☐ Our policies and programs support our health promotion mission.
    ☐ We have strategic priorities for addressing the determinants of health.
    ☐ We value partnerships with diverse organizations and communities.

Culture   ☐ Our leaders and managers enable health promotion practice.
    ☐ We foster critical reflection, innovation, and learning.
    ☐ Health promotion principles and values are practised and celebrated at all levels.
    ☐ Positive and nurturing relationships are fostered among employees.
    ☐ Communication throughout the organization is open and timely.

Structures   ☐ Health promotion is a shared responsibility.
    ☐ Health promotion is integral to our accountability mechanisms.
    ☐ Our structures facilitate collaboration, both internally and externally.
    ☐ We have effective policies for human resource development.
    ☐ We use empowering and evidence-based processes for strategic and program planning.

Resources   ☐ We have many employees with solid knowledge and skills in health promotion.
    ☐ We dedicate adequate human resources to health promotion activities.
    ☐ Resources for health promotion are allocated from our core budget.
    ☐ We actively engage with our communities.
    ☐ We provide practitioners with adequate infrastructure and equipment to do their jobs.

Figure 8.3

Environmental health promotion capacity checklist

Category

Political will	☐ Federal and provincial governments provide adequate financial resources for the comprehensive health system, including care, prevention, and promotion.
	☐ Federal and provincial departments of health provide leadership for the health promotion agenda.
	☐ Regional health care organizations are mandated to invest core funding in population health promotion.
	☐ Governing boards of regional health care organizations value and support health promotion as a core mandate of their organization.
Public opinion	☐ People have a holistic understanding of health and its determinants.
	☐ People believe that addressing the determinants of health is a shared responsibility.
	☐ People take ownership of and responsibility for their own health and well-being.
	☐ People take collective action to foster community well-being.
	☐ People believe that the health system has a mandate for health promotion.
	☐ Positive public and media attention is paid to health promotion.
Supportive organizations	☐ Diverse organizations address the determinants of health.
	☐ Supportive organizations include those from outside the health care sector.
	☐ Supportive organizations frequently partner with one another, including intersectorally.
	☐ Supportive organizations are linked both through informal networks and formal associations.
	☐ Supportive organizations advocate to enhance the credibility of health promotion.
Ideas and other resources	☐ Stimulating and innovative ideas about promoting health are widely accessible.
	☐ Evidence for the effectiveness of health promotion can be easily found.
	☐ Resource materials and conceptual tools are available for a wide range of health promotion strategies, initiatives, and processes.
	☐ Networks of researchers and practitioners are available for advice and support with regard to specific challenges.
	☐ Appropriate opportunities exist for professional development in health promotion.

Figure 8.4

The elements of health promotion capacity

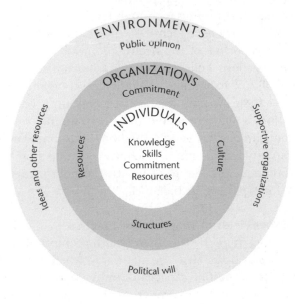

At the organizational level, the seven key catalysts to the development of health promotion capacity are: (1) opportunities for individuals and teams to work on meaningful projects and partnerships, (2) access to resources targeted toward health promotion, (3) planning and evaluation exercises, (4) individual capacity building, (5) changes in key personnel, (6) organizational restructuring, and (7) strategic actions of change agents. These seven catalysts clearly indicate that individuals and the larger environment have a decisive influence on such capacity. The environment itself is subject to change through activities such as advocacy, political action, social movements, capacity building, and the dissemination of research.

Insights for Health Promotion
Our findings offer important insights for people working in health promotion. For health promotion practitioners, we have presented a coherent framework for effective professional practice in the field. Practitioners will take from this book a greater understanding of what health promotion capacity is and how to develop it. For leaders in health sector organizations, we have presented a coherent framework for the

development of organizations that foster and support health promotion action. Leaders will take from this book a greater understanding of how to support health promotion practice, and of how to recruit and develop individual practitioners with high levels of capacity. For health sector policy makers, we have identified the characteristics of environments that are supportive of the health promotion capacity of individuals and organizations. Policy makers will take from this book a greater understanding of how to support individuals and organizations in the development of their capacity for health promotion. For scholars of health promotion, we have proposed an understanding of capacity and its development, and we have established methods of research through which such capacity may be studied. Scholars will take from this book a series of claims about the nature of health promotion capacity and a methodology for exploring such claims.

Insights for Other Fields of Professional Practice
For readers working in fields other than health promotion, our findings have four key implications. First, the manner in which we have conceptualized the health promotion capacity of individuals and organizations may be directly generalizable to other domains of professional practice. Our definition of capacity lends itself to operationalization in a variety of contexts. For individual practitioners, the specific capacities required to work effectively in different places and fields vary considerably. In many contexts, however, capacity to engage in effective professional practice involves some combination of knowledge, skill, commitment, and resources. For organizations in a very broad spectrum of fields, the capacity to foster and support effective professional practices would involve some combination of commitment, culture, structures, and resources. In this way, our conceptualization of capacity provides something of a template that may be applied in other fields. Our work contributes a unique perspective to the literatures of both human resource development and organizational development.

Second, the manner in which we have facilitated the development of capacity among individuals and organizations may be usefully adapted for other fields. Our program planning and instructional methods provide examples for those engaged in continuing professional education, human resource development, and organizational development. Chapters 4 and 5 illustrate that continuing education, practical experience, and critical reflection are the three pillars of intentionally developing the capacity of practitioners and leaders in the field of health promotion. While the substantive content of capacity development would be different in other fields, the educational or transformational process to be facilitated would be relatively similar.

Third, our research methods are replicable in other contexts. Other researchers might usefully follow our three-step approach: (1) begin with a rich understanding of the context of a field of professional practice, (2) work collaboratively with practitioners and organizational leaders to conceptualize and develop measurement procedures regarding the concept of capacity, and (3) engage practitioners and organizational leaders in an extended exploration of their capacity to undertake and support effective professional practice.

Fourth, our findings suggest several useful avenues for future research in the area of capacity for professional practice in fields other than health promotion. What elements of capacity can be generalized to the broadest range of contexts? What elements of capacity have the greatest impact on practice? How do the elements of capacity interact to produce the overall capacity of an individual or an organization? What continuing education activities best enhance capacity to engage in professional practices? What organizational development interventions best enhance an organization's capacity to support professional practice? How do different barriers influence the capacities of practitioners and organizations? How can such barriers be removed or reduced?

In this book, we have explored how individuals become more effective in health promotion work and how organizations become more effective in supporting such work. We organized this exploration around the concept of capacity, and we identified action for learning and learning from action as key processes in capacity-building initiatives. We hope scholars of health promotion and related fields find that the ideas presented in this book provoke further thought and research. We hope practitioners and leaders in these fields find that the ideas presented here provide practical guidance to building the capacity of individuals and organizations. We learned much through working with friends and colleagues on this book, and we hope our readers will find value in the written product of that learning.

References

Advisory Board, International Heart Health Conference. 1992. *The Victoria declaration on heart health*. Victoria, BC, 28 May.

Advisory Board, Second International Heart Health Conference. 1995. *The Catalonia declaration: Investing in heart health*. Barcelona, 1 June.

Advisory Board, Third International Heart Health Conference. 1998. *The Singapore declaration: Forging the will for heart health in the next millennium*. Singapore, 2 September.

Advisory Board, Fourth International Heart Health Conference. 2001. *The Osaka declaration: Health, economics and political action – Stemming the global tide of cardiovascular disease*. Osaka, 27 May.

Advisory Board, Fifth International Heart Health Conference. 2004. *The Milan declaration: Positioning technology to serve global heart health*. Milan, 16 June.

Barnsley, J. 1992. *Research for change: Participatory action research for community groups*. Vancouver: Women's Research Centre.

Basch, C.E., J.D. Eveland, and B. Portnoy. 1986. Diffusion systems for education and learning about health. *Family and Community Health* 9 (2): 1-26.

Berger, P., and T. Luckmann. 1966. *The social construction of reality*. New York: Anchor.

Berkowitz, M. 2000. *An evaluation of Health Promotion Summer School '99*. M.Sc. thesis, University of Saskatchewan.

Bourdieu, P. 1977. *Outline of a theory of practice*. Cambridge: Cambridge University Press.

Bracht, N., ed. 1990. *Health promotion at the community level*. Newbury Park, CA: Sage.

Bracht, N., and A. Tsouros. 1990. Principles and strategies of effective community participation. *Health Promotion International* 5 (3): 199-208.

Brunt, H., B. Reeder, P. Stephenson, E. Love, and Y. Chen. 1995. The Hutterite and Rural Saskatchewan Heart Health Surveys: A comparison of physical and laboratory measures. In *Agricultural health and safety: Workplace, environment, sustainability*, ed. H. McDuffie et al., 513-20. Boca Raton, FL: Lewis.

Butterfoss, F.D., R.M. Goodman, and A. Wandersman. 1993. Community coalitions for prevention and health promotion. *Health Education Research: Theory and Practice* 8 (3): 315-30.

Casebeer, A., C. Scott, and K. Hannah. 2000. Transforming a health care system: Managing change for community gain. *Canadian Journal of Public Health* 91 (2): 89-93.

Chavis, D. 1995. Building community capacity to prevent violence through coalitions and partnerships. *Journal of Health Care for the Poor and Underprivileged* 6 (2): 234-45.

Clark, N., and K. McLeroy. 1995. Creating capacity through health education: What we know and what we don't. *Health Education Quarterly* 22 (3): 273-89.

Commission on the Future of Health Care in Canada. 2002. *Building on values: The future of health care in Canada.* Ottawa: Government of Canada.

Commission on Medicare. 2001. *Caring for medicare: Sustaining a quality system.* Regina: Government of Saskatchewan.

Crisp, B.R., H. Swerissen, and S.J. Duckett. 2000. Four approaches to capacity building in health: Consequences for measurement and accountability. *Health Promotion International* 15 (2): 99-107.

Downie, R., C. Fyfe, and A. Tannahill. 1990. *Health promotion: Models and values.* Oxford: Oxford University Press.

Ebbesen, L.S., B. Reeder, L. Knox, S. Neilson, A. Mansour, and L. Rutherford. 1996. *Community-based cardiovascular disease and stroke prevention in Saskatchewan.* Unpublished manuscript.

Ebbesen, L.S., L. Rutherford, and B. Reeder. 1996. *Heart health promotion: The Saskatchewan story.* Unpublished manuscript.

Elder, J.P., E.S. Geller, M.F. Hovell, and J.A. Mayer. 1994. *Motivating health behavior.* Albany, NY: Delmar Publishers.

Elliott, S.J., M. Taylor, R. Cameron, and R. Schabas. 1998. Assessing public health capacity to support community-based heart health promotion: The Canadian Heart Health Initiative, Ontario Project (CHHIOP). *Health Education Research* 13 (4): 607-22.

Epp, J. 1986. Achieving health for all: A framework for health promotion. *Health Promotion* 1: 419-28.

Evans, R.G., M.L. Barer, and T.R. Marmor, eds. 1994. *Why are some people healthy and others not?* New York: Aldine de Gruyter.

Ewles, L., and I. Simnett. 1992. *Promoting health: A practical guide.* 2nd ed. London: Scutari.

Feather, J. 1994a. Promoting health in Saskatchewan. In *Health promotion in Canada: Provincial, national and international perspectives,* ed. A. Pederson, M. O'Neill, and I. Rootman, 178-94. Toronto: W.B. Saunders.

–. 1994b. *Reflections on health promotion practice.* Saskatoon: University of Saskatchewan, Prairie Region Health Promotion Research Centre.

Feather, J., and B. Sproat. 1996. *Population health promotion: Bringing our visions together.* Conference proceedings. Saskatoon: University of Saskatchewan, Prairie Region Health Promotion Research Centre.

Feather, J., and R. Labonte. 1995. *Sharing knowledge gained from health promotion practice.* Saskatoon: University of Saskatchewan, Prairie Region Health Promotion Research Centre.

Feather, J., V. McGowan, and M. Moore. 1994. *Planning health needs assessment: The basic choices.* Saskatoon: University of Saskatchewan, Prairie Region Health Promotion Research Centre.

Federal, Provincial, and Territorial Advisory Committee on Population Health. 1994. *Strategies for population health: Investing in the health of Canadians.* Ottawa: Minister of Supply and Services Canada.

–. 1999. *Toward a healthy future: Second report on the health of Canadians.* Ottawa: Minister of Supply and Services Canada.

Freudenberg, N., E. Eng, B. Flay, G. Parcel, T. Rogers, and N. Wallerstein. 1995. Strengthening individual and community capacity to prevent disease and promote health: In search of relevant theories and principles. *Health Education Quarterly* 22 (3): 290-306.

Goodman, R.M., and A.B. Steckler. 1990. Mobilizing organizations for health enhancement: Theories of organizational change. In *Health behavior and health education: Theory, research and practice,* ed. K. Glanz, F.M. Lewis, and B.K. Rimer, 314-41. San Francisco: Jossey-Bass.

Goodman, R., M. Speers, K. McLeroy, S. Fawcett, M. Kegler, E. Parker, S. Smith, T. Sterling, and N. Wallerstein. 1998. Identifying and defining the dimensions of community capacity to provide a basis for measurement. *Health Education and Behavior* 25 (3): 258-78.

Green, L.W., L. Richard, and L. Potvin. 1996. Ecological foundations of health promotion. *American Journal of Health Promotion* 10 (4): 270-81.

Green, L.W., and M.W. Kreuter. 1991. *Health promotion planning: An educational and environmental approach.* 2nd ed. Toronto: Mayfield.

Hawe, P., L. King, M. Noort, S. Gifford, and B. Lloyd. 1998. Working invisibly: Health workers talk about capacity-building in health promotion. *Health Promotion International* 13 (4): 285-95.

Hawe, P., M. Noort, L. King, and C. Jordens. 1997. Multiplying health gains: The critical role of capacity-building within health promotion programs. *Health Policy* 39: 29-42.

Health Canada. 1993. *Promoting heart health in Canada: A focus on heart health inequalities.* Ottawa: Minister of Supply and Services Canada.

–. 1998. *Taking action on population health.* Ottawa: Minister of Supply and Services Canada.

Health and Welfare Canada. 1992a. The Canadian Heart Health Initiative. *Health Promotion* 30 (4) (Insert): 1-20.

–. 1992b. *Heart health equality: Mobilizing communities for action.* Ottawa: Minister of Supply and Services Canada.

Holmlund, M. 1998. *A feasibility study on prairie health promotion electronic networking.* Saskatoon: Prairie Region Health Promotion Research Centre.

Israel, B., B. Checkoway, A. Schulz, and M. Zimmerman. 1994. Health education and community empowerment: Conceptualizing and measuring perceptions of individual, organizational, and community control. *Health Education Quarterly* 21 (2): 149-70.

Jackson, T., S. Mitchell, and M. Wright. 1989. The community development continuum. *Community Health Studies* 13 (1): 66-73.

Kang, R. 1995. Building community capacity for health promotion: A challenge for public health nurses. *Public Health Nursing* 12 (5): 312-18.

Kelleher, C. 1996. Education and training in health promotion: Theory and methods. *Health Promotion International* 11 (1): 47-53.

Kirkpatrick, D.L. 1994. *Evaluating training programs: The four levels.* San Francisco: Berrett-Koehler.

Kuyek, J., and R. Labonte. 1995. *Power: Transforming its practices.* Saskatoon: University of Saskatchewan, Prairie Region Health Promotion Research Centre.

Kwan, B., J. Frankish, D. Quantz, and J. Flores. 2003. *A synthesis paper on the conceptualization and measurement of community capacity.* Vancouver: University of British Columbia, Institute of Health Promotion Research.

Labonte, R. 1987. Community health promotion strategies. *Health Promotion* 26 (1): 5-10, 32.

–. 1993a. Community development and partnerships. *Canadian Journal of Public Health* 84 (4): 237-40.

–. 1993b. A holosphere of healthy and sustainable communities. *Australian Journal of Public Health* 17 (1): 4-12.

–. 1993c. *Health promotion and empowerment: Practice frameworks.* Toronto: ParticipACTION.

–. 1994. Health promotion and empowerment: Reflections on professional practice. *Health Education Quarterly* 21 (2): 253-68.

McLean, S.D. 1999. Thinking about research in continuing education: A meta-theoretical primer. *Canadian Journal of University Continuing Education* 25 (2): 23-42.

Miller, D., S. Miller, and S.D. McLean. 1996. *Directory of Saskatchewan self-help groups.* Saskatoon: University of Saskatchewan Extension Press.

Mitchell, C., and L. Sackney. 2000. *Profound improvement: Building capacity for a learning community.* Lisse, NL: Swets and Zeitlinger.

Monahan, J., and M. Scheirer. 1988. The role of linking agents in the diffusion of health promotion programs. *Health Education Quarterly* 15 (4): 417-33.

Orlandi, M.A., C. Landers, R. Weston, and N. Haley. 1990. Diffusion of health promotion innovations. In *Health behavior and health education: Theory, research and practice,* ed. K. Glanz et al., 288-313. San Francisco: Jossey-Bass.

Poole, D.L. 1997. Building community capacity to promote social and public health: Challenges for universities. *Health and Social Work* 22: 163-70.

Raphael, D. 2002. *Social justice is good for our hearts: Why societal factors – not lifestyles – are major causes of heart disease in Canada and elsewhere.* Toronto: CSJ Foundation for Research and Education.

–. 2003. Barriers to addressing the societal determinants of health: Public health units and poverty in Ontario, Canada. *Health Promotion International* 18 (4): 397-405.

Reeder, B. 1990. *Report of the Saskatchewan Heart Health Survey.* Regina: Saskatchewan Health.

Reeder, B., L. Liu, and L. Horlick. 1996. Sociodemographic variation in the prevalence of cardiovascular disease in Saskatchewan: Results from the Saskatchewan Heart Health Survey. *Canadian Journal of Cardiology* 12 (3): 271-77.

Rogers, A. 1993. Adult education and agricultural extension: Some comparisons. *International Journal of Lifelong Education* 12 (3): 165-76.

Rogers, J.M. 1987. *Mutual aid as a mechanism for health promotion and disease prevention.* Health Services and Promotion Branch working paper. Ottawa: Health and Welfare Canada.

Saskatchewan Bureau of Statistics. 1995. *Economic review 1995.* Regina: Saskatchewan Bureau of Statistics.

Saskatchewan Economic Development. 1995. *Regional economic development authorities: Building capacity and sharing responsibility in community-based economic development.* Regina: Saskatchewan Economic Development.

Saskatchewan Education. 2001. *School plus. A vision for children and youth: The final report of the task force and public dialogue on the role of the school: Toward a new school, community and human service partnership in Saskatchewan.* Regina: Saskatchewan Education.

Saskatchewan Health. 1992. *Working together toward wellness: A Saskatchewan vision for health.* Regina: Saskatchewan Health.

–. 2002. *The action plan for Saskatchewan health care.* Regina: Saskatchewan Health.

Saskatchewan Health, Population Health Branch. 1997. *Population health promotion model: A resource binder and supplemental resources.* Regina: Saskatchewan Health.

–. 1999. *A population health promotion framework for Saskatchewan health districts.* Regina: Saskatchewan Health.

Saskatchewan Heart Health Coalition. 1997. Saskatchewan Heart Health Program: II. Demonstration phase. *Saskatchewan Medical Journal* 8 (1): 13-16.

Saskatchewan Heart Health Program. 1998a. *Technical Report 1 – Partnerships.* Saskatoon: University of Saskatchewan.

–. 1998b. *Technical Report 2 – Effective community strategies.* Saskatoon: University of Saskatchewan.

–. 1998c. *Technical Report 3 – Evaluation tools.* Saskatoon: University of Saskatchewan.

–. 1998d. *Technical Report 4 – Dissemination strategies.* Saskatoon: University of Saskatchewan.

–. 1999a. *Tri-District workshop: Evaluation report.* Saskatoon: University of Saskatchewan.

–. 1999b. *Battleford Service Area health promotion workshop: Evaluation report.* Saskatoon: University of Saskatchewan.

–. 2001. *Southeastern Service Area health promotion workshop: Evaluation report.* Saskatoon: University of Saskatchewan.

–. 2002a. *Southwestern Service Area health promotion workshop: Evaluation report.* Saskatoon: University of Saskatchewan.

–. 2002b. *HPLINK. An electronic network discussion group for health promotion: Evaluation report.* Saskatoon: University of Saskatchewan.

–. 2002c. *Building Better Tomorrows conference: Evaluation report.* Saskatoon: University of Saskatchewan.

Saskatchewan Human Services Integration Forum. 2000. *Saskatchewan human services: Working with communities.* Regina: Saskatchewan Human Services Integration Forum.

Saskatchewan Municipal Government. 1993. *Report of the Minister's Advisory Committee on Inter-Community Co-operation and Community Quality of Life.* Regina: Saskatchewan Municipal Government.

–. 1995. *Responding to the community: Proposals for cultural development.* Regina: Saskatchewan Municipal Government.

Saskatchewan Provincial Health Council. 1994. *Population health goals for Saskatchewan.* Regina: Saskatchewan Provincial Health Council.

Schwartz, R., C. Smith, M. Speers, L. Dusenbury, F. Bright, S. Hedlund, F. Wheeler, and T. Schmid. 1993. Capacity building and resource needs of state health agencies to implement community-based cardiovascular disease programs. *Journal of Public Health Policy* 14 (4): 480-94.

Shapiro, M., C. Cartwright, and S. Macdonald. 1994. Community development in primary health care. *Community Development Journal* 29 (3): 222-31.

Simbandumwe, L., M. Fulton, and L. Hammond Ketilson. 1991. *The co-operative sector in Saskatchewan*. Saskatoon: Centre for the Study of Co-operatives.

Smith, D. 1990. *The conceptual practices of power: A feminist sociology of knowledge*. Toronto: University of Toronto Press.

Smith, N., B. Littlejohns, and D. Thompson. 2001. Shaking out the cobwebs: Insights into community capacity and its relation to health outcomes. *Community Development Journal* 36 (1): 30-41.

Stabler, J., M. Olfert, and M. Fulton. 1992. *The changing role of rural communities in an urbanizing world: Saskatchewan 1961-1990*. Regina: Canadian Plains Research Centre.

Stachenko, S. 1996. The Canadian Heart Health Initiative: A countrywide cardiovascular disease prevention strategy. *Journal of Human Hypertension* 10 (1): S.5-S.8.

Tones, K., and S. Tilford. 1994. *Health education: Effectiveness, efficacy and equity*. 2nd ed. London: Chapman and Hall.

Wallack, L. 1994. Media advocacy: A strategy for empowering people and communities. *Journal of Public Health Policy* 2: 420-36.

World Health Organization. 1986. The Ottawa charter for health promotion. *Health Promotion* 1: iii-v.

Index

Note: "(f)" following a page number indicates a figure, "(t)" indicates a table. BHPC stands for Building Health Promotion Capacity project; HPC, for Health Promotion Contact; PRHPRC, for Prairie Region Health Promotion Research Centre; SHHP, for Saskatchewan Heart Health Program; SPHPP, for Saskatchewan Population Health Promotion Partnership.